Inspiring and Supporting Behavior Change

A Food, Nutrition, and Health Professional's Counseling Guide

Second Edition

Cecilia Sauter, MS, RD, CDE, FAADE

Ann Constance, MA, RD, CDE, FAADE

eat right.® **Academy of Nutrition and Dietetics**

Inspiring and Supporting Behavior Change: A Food, Nutrition, and Health Professional's Counseling Guide, Second Edition

ISBN 978-0-88091-982-1 print

ISBN 978-0-88091-993-8 eBook

Catalog Number 455617, 455617e

For more information on the Academy of Nutrition and Dietetics, visit www.eatright.org.

Reviewers

Judy Dowd, MA, RD, LDN
Director of the University of Massachusetts
Dietetic Internship
Amherst, MA

Carolyn Harrington, RD, LDN, CDE
Independent Contractor
Venice, FL

Angela Lemond, RD, CSP, LD
Owner, Lemond Nutrition
Plano, TX

Erin Rigney, MS, RD
Nutrition Education Supervisor
Round Rock, TX

Contents

Foreword

Congratulations on choosing this book! I am so pleased to introduce you to the second edition of this wonderful resource, and I know that you will find it helpful in your practice and for your patients.

Chronic illnesses such as diabetes require considerable effort for patients, their families, and health care professionals. Patients and their families are often asked to adjust eating habits and choice of foods, lose weight, become more physically active, monitor health indicators such as blood pressure and blood glucose levels, take multiple medications, and perform other self-care activities throughout the day. In addition to lifestyle changes, patients need to cope with the emotional impact and distress of a chronic illness that can result in multiple complications and premature death. Self-management involves incorporating the many day-to-day decisions this entails while still managing all of the other priorities in their already complex and stressful lives. While technology, new medications, and other treatment methodologies offer hope for a healthier future, they often increase the demands on patients in terms of time, problem-solving, thought, and effort.

One of the realities of all chronic illnesses is that the patient is ultimately responsible for implementing the treatment plan. This responsibility is based on three characteristics: choices, control, and consequences. The lifestyle and therapeutic choices patients make each day directly affect their outcomes. In addition, patients are in charge and control of their self-management choices and behaviors. We can provide information and create an effective plan, but it is completely up to the patient to decide if they will implement some or all of these recommendations or ignore or reject our advice. While frustrating for health professionals, self-management of chronic illnesses belongs to patients and their families because the positive and negative consequences of the daily decisions accrue first and foremost to them.

Self-management education and ongoing support is essential for behavior change. This education needs to include not only "what to do" but also "why it needs to occur," such as the potential short- and long-term consequences. However, because of the number and complexity of lifestyle changes, most adults need additional information and ongoing support to make and sustain the behaviors required for a lifetime of self-management. We need to not only educate patients about the "what and why" of behavior change but also teach *how* to make those changes, how to maintain them for a lifetime of chronic illness, and, most importantly, how to effectively cope with the emotional demands and distress of their illness.

As in the first edition of this book, Ann and Cecilia have created a comprehensive resource and guide. It provides current, evidence-based information about how to help patients who are working to make lifestyle changes and how various approaches and strategies can be used in different situations. Major changes in this edition include additional information about effective strategies such as empowerment-based education and goal setting and motivational interviewing. The findings of the groundbreaking international DAWN2 about the psychosocial impact and burden of diabetes and diabetes-related distress on patients and families are included, as are additional strategies for ongoing support, the best use of technology, and peer supporters. In addition, a new chapter includes meditation and other strategies for coping with the competing demands and stress of daily life.

In short, this book gives you the tools you need to be an effective registered dietitian as you work with patients who have diabetes or another chronic condition. With your help through the strategies delineated in this book, they make informed choices, take control, and achieve improved outcomes as a consequence of their efforts.

Martha M. Funnell, MS, RN, CDE, FAADE
Associate Research Scientist
Department of Learning Health Sciences
University of Michigan Medical School
Ann Arbor, MI

Chapter 1:
Oh, No! Don't Tell Me
I Have to Change!

Nobody likes change except a baby in wet diapers.

In a perfect world, our patients would always be motivated to follow our recommendations. Once they leave our offices, they would immediately implement the meal plan ideas we presented. They'd start being more physically active. They'd even start eating whole grains! As they moved toward their health goals, they would begin seeing results and, before long, they'd send us bouquets of "thank you" flowers. Of course, we live in the real world, and we know that human behavior is more complex than that.

Bob's Story

Take Bob, for example. Bob is 65 years old, has poorly controlled type 2 diabetes, and weighs almost 300 pounds. In addition, his blood pressure, cholesterol, and triglycerides are too high; his HDL cholesterol is only 28 mg/dL; and he is taking several medications. Bob's doctor referred him to a registered dietitian nutritionist (RDN), Susan, to help learn how to make changes to his eating habits, which will assist with weight loss and getting his blood glucose, lipids, and pressure under better control.

At Bob's first appointment, Susan weighs and measures him. She also asks several questions about his current level of physical activity and how often he eats out each week. Then she calculates the number of calories Bob needs to consume each day to begin losing weight slowly (1 to 2 pounds per week) and develops a meal plan for him based on that number. For the remainder of the appointment, Susan and Bob go over the suggested meal plan, and Susan offers plenty of advice about what to eat. She uses food models to teach Bob about portion control. She also gives Bob a comprehensive "eating out" handout to take home. If he follows these instructions, he should begin to see results!

Bob never follows the great advice from this trained nutrition expert. He is used to skipping breakfast, often missing lunch, and then eating a big dinner and grazing for the rest of the evening. In contrast, Susan designed a plan that included three meals and an evening snack each day. To Bob, this meal plan seems overwhelming and unacceptable. He feels like he's being asked to make many changes at once, and most of the changes involve things he has been doing for many years. In addition, he does not really see the benefit in making these changes. As is too often the case in the health care arena, Bob fails to keep his follow-up appointment with Susan.

Reaching the "Unreachable" Patient

What went wrong? Are patients like Bob "unreachable"? Are they destined for the noncompliant/no-show section of our file drawer or for the "inactive patients" file in our computer database? Could Susan, the RDN, have done things differently to help Bob identify changes he was willing to make and follow through with?

How many of your patients secretly dread that you are going to make them stop eating all of their favorite foods? How many splurge the day or week before seeing you, anticipating that their favorite foods will soon be "forbidden"? How many think they will have to give up foods that taste good because the foods cannot be healthy for them? Perhaps they expect they will be eating nothing but lettuce, broccoli, and high-fiber cereal for the rest of their lives. Whether your patients have diabetes, kidney disease, obesity, or any number of other health conditions, these thoughts are probably going through their minds.

We know nutrition and exercise are just as important as medication to improve or maintain health, but many patients find changes to their food and activity habits much more difficult than taking medication. And, frankly, they may not *want* to change, or they may not realize how crucial these modifications are to their health.

RDNs face such challenges every day. That's why we wrote this book—to give you the tools and know-how to inspire patients to take control and manage lifestyle changes for better health. In addition to your clinical knowledge, you can learn to become an effective change agent!

How we approach and support our patients can be critical to whether or not they successfully make difficult lifestyle changes. As a trained food and nutrition expert, you have a lot of great advice to share with your patients. What you may need to learn is *how* and *when* to share that expertise. If knowledge were the single most important thing we needed to share with patients, we would have thousands of reformed eaters in our communities. Our friends, family members, and coworkers would be "perfect eaters" too! In addition, no one would smoke, and all of us would get at least 120 minutes of physical activity each week.

Success Is All in the Approach

It is not necessary to change. Survival is not mandatory.

—*W. Edwards Deming*

In Bob's case, he received enough education. Susan certainly gave him the *information* he needed to make lifestyle changes. Bob, however, lacked the *desire* to change and *confidence* to follow through on the proposed changes.

In this book, we will teach you how to be more successful when counseling patients. We will discuss ways to help patients identify what is most important to them, to work with them to set goals, and to enhance their confidence in making the changes. We will show you how to wrap up patient visits by collaborating to make a plan that is important to them, identifying one thing they think they can complete over the course of the next week or two.

The process of figuring out what the patient really wants and feels willing to do might take skills you haven't fully developed in the classroom or continuing education programs. In this book, you will learn ways to identify a patient's willingness to change. We will also show you how to use strategies like empowerment to help guide patients toward making their own behavior change plans, which they will be more likely to implement.

We discuss how to form partnerships with patients and help empower them to take charge of their lives and lifestyle changes. We explain how to help patients look at their options for change as well as the consequences of not making these adjustments. And we demonstrate the value of supporting patients in making small improvements as well as large ones—over time, baby steps can add up to a *big* change!

Reading this book can also help you hone your listening skills. We discuss communication techniques, like reflective listening, that will enhance your patients' willingness to change.

Paul's Story: Similar Situation, Different Result

Insanity: Doing the same thing over and over again and expecting different results.

—*Albert Einstein*

If your patients are not making changes or are not coming back for follow-up appointments, perhaps it is time for *you* to try a different approach. In that light, let's turn to Paul's story.

Paul is an avid hunter in the Upper Peninsula of Michigan, who shares many of the same health concerns as Bob. He is in his sixties, has had poorly controlled diabetes for many years, and, like Bob, is overweight, has elevated blood pressure and abnormal lipids, and takes many medications. Paul also recently had coronary bypass surgery. Unfortunately, the incision on his lower leg is not healing, and he is at risk for having his leg amputated.

The opening day of deer hunting season is coming up. Paul looks forward to meeting his friends at hunting camp every year. He is motivated to do anything to save his leg and make it to hunting camp this year. Taking his doctor's advice, Paul makes an appointment with an RDN, Irene, for medical nutrition therapy.

During the first encounter, Irene spends time getting to know Paul in order to understand what is important to him. She asks why he came for nutrition counseling today and what his greatest concern is. Paul replies that he wants his leg to heal so he can hunt. Their conversation then turns to what Paul already knows about diabetes, controlling diabetes, and how diabetes is linked to wound healing. Guided by pertinent questions from Irene, Paul identifies a couple of changes he is willing to make while still keeping his focus on the prize—going to hunting camp.

Irene recognizes that Paul needs to decide what *he* wants to work on and helps him set a goal to accomplish over the next 1 to 2 weeks. Before the session ends, Irene checks to make sure that Paul has a high level of confidence to follow through on the action steps he set for himself. Luckily, Paul has also brought a support person to the visit, his wife, Jan. Her participation is important because she does most of the grocery shopping and cooking. Over the next couple of weeks, Paul is indeed motivated to take action, and his blood glucose levels improve. He returns for his follow-up appointments, too. If his health continues to improve, he can focus on what he truly enjoys—his hunting trips.

It should be clear why Paul was able to meet his goals but Bob wasn't. In Paul's case, RDN Irene focused on his motivations for seeking medical nutrition therapy. In Bob's case, RDN Susan never found out much about him, his likes and interests, or his motivations. She also didn't find out what Bob already knew about diabetes. Susan directed their conversation and presented him with changes to make, rather than involving Bob in the process.

Forming Relationships

As the stories of Bob and Paul illustrate, developing rapport is key when working with patients. However, for some RDNs, the ability to form relationships may not come naturally. It might help to think of your role as that of a salesperson. Successful salespeople listen to what people want and build trust with their customers. You can use similar techniques to identify patient concerns and priorities during nutrition counseling. The successful "sale" for the RDN comes when the patient sets a goal and achieves it!

What's Next?

This book focuses primarily on the work you do with your patients on an individual basis. However, your patients may also have a difficult time making and sustaining behavior change because the health system is not set up to effectively help patients with chronic health care conditions. Chapter 2, therefore, discusses some of the challenges that you and your patients may encounter in the health care system and in the community, as well as solutions that institutions, communities, and individual RDNs can seek.

In Chapters 3 through 6, you will find tips and techniques for helping patients identify what is most important to them regarding health goals. More specifically, Chapter 3 looks at empowering patients, Chapter 4 covers the stages of change model of behavior change, and Chapter 5 explains motivational interviewing. In Chapter 6, we put these strategies together as we guide you through processes that will help you assist your patients to set reasonable, self-selected goals—goals they will take ownership of, not react to.

Throughout this book, you'll find examples of how emotions can affect patients' desire and ability to change. One of the authors of this book met a man with diabetes who compared his experiences of living with diabetes to when he was diagnosed with and treated for colon cancer. He said the negative emotions associated with diabetes management were *more* pronounced than the negative emotions surrounding his cancer diagnosis and treatment. During his cancer treatment, this man had a fairly passive role—once the appropriate treatment was determined, he just "sat back" and let the health care professionals perform surgery and administer chemotherapy. At every visit related to his cancer treatment, the medical staff checked on his mental and emotional health, too. With diabetes, *he* had to make and carry out most of the decisions—what to eat, how much insulin to take, when to check his blood glucose, and what to do if his glucose levels went too high or too low.[1] Unfortunately, his diabetes care providers did not check on or provide assistance for diabetes distress or anxiety. Chapter 7 explores further the effect of diabetes distress and offers advice about working with patients who may need emotional or mental health support as well as treatment for serious health problems. The chapter addresses ways to identify patients who may have emotional/mental health issues like anxiety and depression, and how to refer them for additional care when their needs go beyond the scope of your practice. This chapter also includes guidance on financial resources for patients whose adherence with treatment may be affected by economic constraints. Chapter 8 provides additional tools and techniques like meditation, deep breathing, and positive thinking that can help patients better deal with health distress and anxiety.

In Chapter 9, we discuss the topic of building long-term support for behavior change. Options for professional and peer support are surveyed. Chapter 10 examines a number of communication-related issues that can affect your counseling abilities—health literacy of patients, cultural and ethnic diversity, and a variety of potential biases that may shape your perspective. The book also includes an appendix of resources for RDNs seeking further information.

Building Self-Efficacy

Throughout the book we present tools and techniques that help build the self-efficacy of your patients. Having a high level of self-efficacy means that a person has the self-belief and confidence to make lifestyle changes. A highly developed self-efficacy also helps give people the confidence to deal with change and new tasks. If they experience difficulty or failure, they are quick to recover and move forward. On the other hand, people with a low self-efficacy may avoid any tasks that seem difficult. They tend to half-heartedly commit to goals and often have a difficult time rebounding from setbacks.[2]

Some of the ways we can help our patients develop their self-efficacy include the following:

- Modeling—If patients see or hear about a peer accomplishing something, it helps give them confidence that they can do the same: "If Joe can do it, I can do it too!"
- Social persuasion—When you or the peers of your patients confidently tell a patient that he or she has the ability to accomplish something, the patient is more likely to be successful.
- Experiences that develop mastery—This is where goal setting is critical. Helping patients set goals that they are confident they can achieve helps them over time master behavior changes that once seemed overwhelming.

When you inspire and support behavior change, you set up a win-win-win situation. First, patients feel good when they are successful. Also, you are excited about no longer being the "bad guy" or feeling that you bear most of the responsibility for patient change—change is in the hands of each patient, and they are setting and accomplishing their health behavior goals. Finally, the health care provider loves seeing health improvements, especially in patients who were once labeled as being noncompliant or resistant to change.

Practice Exercises

Exercise 1

Think about your patients and ask yourself the following questions:

- What percentage of your patients come back for follow-up care?
- How many patients are setting and achieving goals? How many are also improving health parameters?
- How many of your patients would you label as "noncompliant"?

Exercise 2

Now, think about yourself and your own personal health habits and answer the following questions:

- Have you been thinking about changing any of your own health habits?
- Have you taken action on these changes?
- If so, have you been successful? What helped you make the changes?
- If not, why not? What are the barriers you are facing?

References

1. Weiss MA, Funnell MM. *The Little Diabetes Book You Need to Read*. Philadelphia, PA: Running Press; 2007.

2. Bandura A. *Self efficacy*. http://www.uky.edu/~eushe2 /Bandura/BanEncy.html. Accessed June 13, 2015.

Chapter 2:
Patients Change... When We Change: The Patient-Centered Medical Home

Everyone thinks of changing the world, but no one thinks of changing himself.

—Leo Tolstoy

In Chapter 1 we introduced you to Bob and Paul, two men with similar health challenges, including diabetes and overweight, who responded very differently to their encounters with RDNs. Bob disregarded the advice of his RDN and never returned for follow-up. In contrast, Paul succeeded in making changes and demonstrated a willingness to engage in follow-up nutrition counseling. As we sought to explain the different outcomes, we attributed Paul's greater success to the approach his RDN used, which emphasized listening to his needs and interests and helping him set goals based on his personal priorities, such as his desire to go to hunting camp.

Neither of these stories mentioned the training or resources available to the RDNs, the health care systems in which they worked, or the characteristics of the surrounding communities. How might these types of factors contribute to the opportunities for patients to achieve personal success? That question is addressed in this chapter. In particular, we examine the distinctions between acute and chronic health care and explore the components of a model of health care focused on the management of chronic health conditions. As we shall show, system-wide implementation of the patient-centered medical home (PCMH) and the use of the chronic care model (CCM) and the primary care model (PCM) can support the individual efforts of RDNs and other clinicians to improve patient outcomes.

The Scope of Chronic Health Care Demands

Historically, the health care system in the United States was set up to primarily treat *acute* (short-duration) medical problems. For example, a patient would visit a physician when he or she had an illness like pneumonia or an injury like a broken leg. In those cases, the physician was regarded as the expert, and the patient's role was limited and mostly passive, relying on the recommendations of the doctor.

Today, many patient visits to the health care provider are related to *chronic* conditions, such as diabetes, heart disease, or arthritis. According to estimates from the Institute of Medicine,[1] 134 million Americans will have a chronic condition in 2020. Other sources estimate that 80% of outpatient care is linked to providing support for chronic or lifelong illnesses like type 1 and type 2 diabetes, obesity, or heart disease.[2] In 2012, the United States spent $2.8 trillion on health care, and chronic illness accounted for 84% of the spending in 2006.[3] In 2010, total spending for the Medicare population (largely aged ≥ 65 years) was more than $300 billion, and 93% of Medicare spending was for people with two or more chronic conditions.[4]

Supporting Self-Management

> *The name of the game is taking care of yourself because you're going to live long enough to wish you had.*
>
> —Grace Mirabella

In contrast to traditional administration of acute medical care, most care for chronic disease is usually done by the patient between appointments (self-management), while the health care provider's role has shifted to a more passive one, similar to that of a coach or adviser.[5] The reality of a chronic disease is that the patient has the right and the responsibility to make self-management decisions on a daily basis. As Bodenheimer and colleagues explain:[6]

> *Self-management* is what people do every day: they decide what to eat, whether or not to exercise, if and when they will monitor their health, or whether or not they will take their medications. Everyone self-manages, even the patient who chooses *not* to take care of himself. So the question becomes whether or not the choices made will improve their health-related behaviors and therefore lead them to improve their clinical outcomes.

Unfortunately, while the demands of chronic diseases on the health care system have increased greatly, the training of many health care professionals is still based on the older paradigm of dealing with acute illness, where active patient participation is less important. In general, health care providers have not been adequately prepared to deal with chronic conditions, and many health care and community organizations lack systems and programs to treat and support people with chronic health issues.[7,8] Adopting strategies to support the self-management efforts of our patients will enhance our interactions with them and minimize everyone's frustration.

There are three fundamental aspects of chronic care: choices, control, and consequences. Patients make choices every day, that is, whether they take their medication, what they eat, and if they exercise. These choices have a greater impact on their health than any recommendations that the health care provider can give during a single encounter. Also, patients are in charge of their own lives. They decide which recommendations given to them they will follow and which ones they will ignore. Finally, because patients are the ones who make the decisions that best fit into their lives, they are also responsible for the consequences of their decisions.[7,9,10] Many of us may have to fight the urge to try to "fix" our patients—after all, we feel we have so much knowledge and advice to offer that we know our patients would benefit greatly from following our advice!

Self-management in chronic disease usually requires multiple lifestyle changes. However, many health care providers believe they know best which changes the patient needs to make, and they therefore tell the patient how, where, and when to make these lifestyle changes. These providers believe that their expertise in the treatment of the disease also makes them the "expert" of what changes will help the patient the most, regardless of the patient's desires or interests. However, when we ignore or downplay our patients' concerns and priorities, patients feel our recommendations are intrusive, and they may not be ready or able to follow our advice, or our advice might not even be realistic with their lifestyle. This can also lead to providers feeling frustrated because they cannot get their patients to follow their recommendations. These patients are often called "noncompliant."[10]

If this sounds familiar to you, you are not alone. Studies have demonstrated that as many as 50% of patients don't follow long-term medication regimens, more than 80% don't follow advice to change health behaviors, and 20% to 30% don't complete curative medication regimens.[11,12] These statistics may be startling, but they indicate that we need to look at different ways to help our patients help themselves!

When we use good communication skills, more patients are able to follow our recommendations and improve self-care. In these situations, patients are more satisfied with their care and have better health outcomes. In short, to improve outcomes, we must collaborate with patients and encourage their participation in treatment decisions.[13] As an RDN, you are the expert in nutrition, but your patients are the experts in knowing what does and what does not work for them and what they are willing to try. We need to learn to work in partnership with our patients.

The Patient-Centered Medical Home

As an individual RDN, you can do a great deal to strengthen your counseling skills to inspire and support behavior change by your patients (see Chapters 3 through 10). Identifying ways to improve care of patients with chronic conditions may enhance your opportunities for success, and working in a patient-centered medical home

(PCMH) can be a way to assist and help patients with one or multiple chronic conditions.

The PCMH has been around for many years, starting in the pediatric community in the 1960s. Physician shortages and the increase in health care costs have made the concept of the PCMH an attractive one. PCMH combines the frameworks of two very distinct concepts: the primary care model and the chronic care model.

The primary care model (PCM) focuses on the patient and emphasizes whole-person care instead of single-disease-oriented care. The PCM identifies four specific elements: accessibility; a continuous relationship with patients over time; comprehensive care that meets most of the patients' health care needs; and coordination of care across a patient's conditions, providers, and settings.[14]

The chronic care model (CCM), which is a very important aspect of the patient-centered medical home, focuses on strengthening chronic illness management within the primary care setting. Ed Wagner, MD, MPH, and his team at the MacColl Institute at Group Health Cooperative in Seattle, with funding from the Robert Wood Johnson Foundation, developed the CCM. The six elements of the CCM are patient self-management support, clinical information systems, delivery system redesign, decision support, health care organization, and community resources. The chronic care model assumes that each patient with a chronic disease has a primary care physician who coordinates his or her care—that is, has a solid platform of primary care.[15]

The CCM places the responsibility for self-management with the affected individual, while also emphasizing the importance of structured self-management support activities and systems within communities to facilitate healthy behavior changes. According to the CCM, health outcomes improve when an informed and activated patient works with a health care team that is prepared and trained to be proactive and collaborative.[8] An empowered and activated patient may stimulate the clinician to move into action in a partnership type of a relationship, while clinicians (including RDNs) who are trained to be patient centered and collaborative are more likely to empower and engage their patients.

In addition to the patient and his or her team of health care providers, the health care system is a large component of the CCM. Part of the CCM's goal is to create a culture within health care delivery organizations that prioritizes patient care, whether it is chronic or acute in nature, as well as the necessary mechanisms to promote safe and high-quality care for patients.[14]

Recognizing the benefits and evidence behind the primary care model's four key elements, the physician societies added aspects of the CCM to develop the joint principles of the patient-centered medical home in 2007. These principles are shown in Figure 2.1 (page 22).

- Continuity of care—Each patient has an ongoing relationship with a personal physician. The care the patient receives over time is patient focused and not disease specific.

- Coordination of care—The PCMH coordinates all the care the patient receives from other providers (specialists, hospitals, labs, radiology, and so on) to assure that patients get the indicated care when and where they need and want it, including medication review and management.

Figure 2.1: Joint principles of the patient-centered medical home

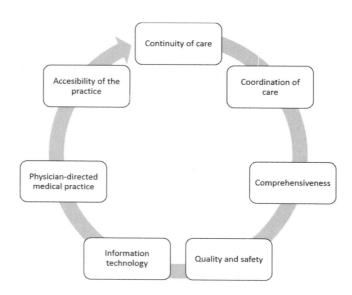

- Comprehensiveness—The PCMH provides care for all stages of life, including acute care, chronic care, preventive services, and end-of-life care. Important elements that are found here include, but are not limited to, planned visits and population health management utilizing patient registries as well as a range of services offered by the PCMH.

  ○ A well-designed delivery system ensures that patients receive effective, efficient clinical care, as well as appropriate self-management support. It is critical that the design consider health literacy and cultural sensitivity (see Chapter 10). Within this system, we can include planned patient visits or group visits for diabetes or other chronic health conditions, as well as clinical case management services for patients with complex health issues. An appropriate health care delivery system will refer patients to RDNs for care or follow-up. As an RDN, you can assist with care management, too.

° Self-management support empowers and prepares patients to manage their health and care. Effective self-management support strategies include appropriate assessment, setting goals, action planning, problem solving, and follow-up. You cannot possibly be the sole or main support person or resource for all of your patients. Seek out internal and community resources that will provide ongoing self-management support to patients. Help link them to the type of support that works best for them. These effort will also enhance patient success.

• Quality and safety—This principle includes several elements from the CCM: decision support, quality-improvement efforts, making sure to include the patients as part of the decision-making process, and getting feedback from the patient to make sure his or her expectations are met.

° Decision support refers to information that promotes clinician care that is consistent with scientific evidence and patient preferences. It integrates evidence-based guidelines with daily clinical practice, making it possible to share evidence-based information with patients, which may encourage their participation in self-care. For instance, when you explain the "ABCs" of diabetes care (ie, hemoglobin A1C, blood pressure, cholesterol control) to a patient and provide information about how to attain those goals, you can help the patient become more proactive in his or her own care. As a result, he or she will know what the desirable health goals are and be aware of the changes needed to attain those goals.

○ Using evidence-based care also helps all members of the health care team stay on the same track. For example, a doctor who writes orders for a 1,000- or 1,200-calorie diet for all patients with diabetes is not practicing evidence-based or patient-centered care. In fact, practices like this can be counterproductive and unreasonable, resulting in patients giving up on making changes because the recommendations are too onerous. Such patients may never return to you for follow-up and may limit their visits to other providers as well. In such situations, patients may not feel better and may be at higher risk for complications if they do not seek medical care. Then the health care system (and taxpayers) must take care of costly complications, many of which could have been prevented through good self-care. Finally, the health care provider is affected with concern and frustration for patients who are "noncompliant."

- Information technology (IT)—The health care system uses IT appropriately to support optimal patient care, performance measurement, patient education, and enhanced communication. Here we find the patient registries that facilitate disease management, population health, and evidence-based care.
    - A clinician information system organizes patient data to facilitate efficient and effective care. For example, a registry of all the patients who have diabetes within an institution helps to track their care and outcomes. Such a registry facilitates the planning of individual patient care and makes it possible to share information with patients and providers, coordinate care, and improve outcomes. How does this benefit the RDN? The registry could identify patients who would benefit from medical nutrition therapy, and their records could be flagged to ensure they receive a referral to an RDN.

- Physician-directed medical practice—This involves a team that "takes collective responsibility for ongoing care of patients," thus ensuring that the increasingly complex needs of patients with multiple chronic conditions are met.[14] Teamwork can facilitate comprehensiveness and coordination of care.
- Accessibility of the practice—The PCMH is a point of entry into the health care system every time new care is needed.[14]

Clearly, RDNs play a role in this part of the PCMH. Even if you are in private practice, you must often coordinate patient care with other team members associated with one or more health care systems. For example, your ability to provide optimal care depends on a health care system that allows you to:

- identify patients who have not received their routine care or have missed their follow-up appointments with other members of the health care team, and
- access patients' health parameters (such as laboratory test results, data from examinations, and health status) that are relevant to the scope of practice of the RDN.

Implementing the Patient-Centered Medical Home

> *All governments must be prepared to deal with the infectious diseases because they could be overwhelming this year or next, but the long-term problem is with the chronic diseases.*
>
> —*Robert Beaglehole, director of the Department of Chronic Disease and Health Promotion, World Health Organization, 2003–2007*

The PCMH is an evidence-based approach. When all or some of the components are implemented, the model supports your patients in setting and achieving their goals. Let us therefore explore how to implement the PCMH within health care institutions.

According to the Institute of Medicine,[1] multiple changes are needed to make our health care system support chronic care management. Detailed information about how health care systems can enhance chronic care management is available on the Making System Changes for Better Diabetes Care website.[16] RDNs employed by health care organizations may be part of chronic care management teams and can also play a role in system redesign. This website offers resources that can help with needed system changes.

You can help to implement evidence-based care in your health care system. When all team members and patients share a consistent approach and objectives, patients are less confused.[16] Look for opportunities to be part of guideline-implementation teams for your health care system, especially for guidelines linked to the RDN scope of practice. For example, some health care systems may use electronic medical records with embedded clinical guidelines, and perhaps you can help review or adapt these guidelines to fit the needs of the organization. Other health care systems may need to go through a formal process to develop, implement, and review guidelines that are evidence based and will be used by all health care team members. You may be able to participate in the following parts of the process:

- putting together a guideline-development team,
- looking at existing evidence-based guidelines already in place and recent research on the issue,
- customizing guidelines based on research and the needs of a particular facility,
- identifying ways to integrate guideline use,
- assessing guideline use, and
- planning regular reviews and revisions.

Ideally, once guidelines are developed, they are supported by automated clinical information and decision support systems through electronic medical records. With electronic medical records, you can access evidence-based guidelines that other team members use in patient treatment. When appropriate, you can then help reinforce guidelines with patients and/or contact another provider when additional care is indicated. For example, if you note that a patient with diabetes has not had a dilated eye exam in more than a year, you could explore that with him or her. Perhaps the patient is unaware of the guidelines for eye exams in diabetes care, or he or she might face other barriers to eye care that the health care team has not addressed.

Similarly, the electronic medical record can also identify for other team members the latest and greatest findings on nutrition interventions. For example, as RDNs, we know that there is no "one size fits all" diet for people with diabetes. With our patients, we collaboratively develop personalized meal plans based on patient goals, preferences, glucose control, and other comorbidities. When the evidence-based guidelines for diabetes meal planning are disseminated to other health care professionals, they can reinforce the recommendations and diminish the use of fad diets. Therefore, RDNs should be involved in guideline development for health care systems or participate in the review of guidelines already implemented.

In addition to participating in the integration of evidence-based guidelines into your health care system, you can also improve chronic care by advocating for systemic support for patient-centered care. Well-planned communication channels through regular team meetings and information technology are one essential step, as it is critical to coordinate patient care in various settings over time.[1]

As you counsel patients, you will want to adjust your approach based on their personal ability to set and achieve goals, but you will also want to consider the structure of the health care system, as well as the availability of other support systems within the community and in the health care system. This process is a bit like juggling several balls at once. It involves more than just working with patients; you also help implement the recommendations of the PCMH on a system- and community-wide basis.

Practice Exercises

Exercise 1

List the various health care system or community resources you currently coordinate patient care with. Are there any types of resources that are needed?

Exercise 2

If you work with or in a health care system, are there parts of the patient-centered medical home that are not already in place that you can help implement? If so, what are they, and what steps will you take to make these changes?

References

1. Committee on Quality of Health Care in America, Institute of Medicine. *Crossing the Quality Chasm: A New Health System for the 21st Century.* Washington, DC: National Academies Press; 2001. http://books.nap.edu/openbook.php?record _id=10027. Accessed June 18, 2015.

2. Grumbach K, Bodenheimer T. A primary care home for Americans: putting the house in order. *JAMA.* 2002;288:889-893.

3. Centers for Disease Control and Prevention. Chronic disease prevention and health promotion. http://www.cdc.gov /chronicdisease/overview/index.htm#sec3. Accessed May 13, 2015.

4. Centers for Medicare and Medicaid Services. *Chronic Conditions Among Medicare Beneficiaries, Chart Book 2012.* Baltimore, MD: Centers for Medicare & Medicaid Services; 2012. http://www.cms.gov/Research-Statistics-Data-and -Systems/Statistics-Trends-and-Reports/Chronic-Conditions /Downloads/2012Chartbook.pdf. Accessed May 13, 2015.

5. Heisler M. Helping your patient with chronic disease: effective physician approaches to support self-management. *Semin Med Pract.* 2005;8:43-54.

6. Bodenheimer T, MacGregor K, Sharifi C. Helping patients manage their chronic conditions. http://www.chcf.org /publications/2005/06/helping-patients-manage-their -chronic-conditions. Published June 2005. Accessed June 18, 2015.

7. Funnell M, Anderson R. Empowerment and self-management of diabetes. *Clin Diabetes.* 2004;22:123-127.

8. Bodenheimer T, Loring K, Holman H, Grumbach K. Patient self-management of chronic disease in primary care. *JAMA.* 2002;288:2469-2475.

9. Glasgow RE, Anderson RM. In diabetes care, moving from compliance to adherence is not enough: something entirely different is needed [letter]. *Diabetes Care.* 1999;22:2090-2092.

10. Rubin RR, Anderson RM, Funnell MM. Collaborative diabetes care. *Pract Diabetol*. 2002;21:29-32.

11. Meichenbaum D, Turk DC. *Facilitating Treatment Adherence: A Practitioner's Guidebook*. New York, NY: Plenum; 1987.

12. DiMatteo MR. Enhancing patient adherence to medical recommendations. *JAMA*. 1994;271:29.

13. Funnell MM, Anderson RM. The problem with compliance in diabetes. *JAMA*. 2000;284:1709.

14. Center for Studying Health System Change. Making medical homes work: moving from concept to practice. *Policy Perspective*. 2008;1:1-20. http://www.pcmh.ahrq.gov/sites/default/files/attachments/Making%20Medical%20Home%20Work_Moving%20from%20Concept%20to%20Practice.pdf. Accessed June 12, 2015.

15. Wagner EH. Chronic disease management: what will it take to improve care for chronic illness? *Eff Clin Pract*. 1998;1:2-4.

16. National Diabetes Education Program, National Institutes of Health. Practice transformation for physicians and health care teams. http://betterdiabetescare.nih.gov. Accessed June 18, 2015.

Chapter 3:
Empowerment: Your Patients in the Driver's Seat

As we discussed in Chapter 2, the choices that patients make every day will have a much larger impact on chronic disease outcomes than any decision the health care providers make during the medical appointments. Patients' choices will affect how they live and the outcome of their diseases. Therefore, patients are responsible not only for their decisions but also for managing their disease.[1-3] The challenge for RDNs and other health care professionals is to provide care that empowers patients to make choices and follow through on behavior change. In that light, let's consider Jeff's and Ana's stories.

Jeff's Story

Jeff is the CEO of a large corporation. He gets his annual health exam at one of the most renowned clinics in the area. During his most recent exam, he was told that his blood pressure was elevated and he also has diabetes. Jeff met with a nurse who explained how to monitor his blood glucose and with an RDN who provided instruction on how to modify his diet and lose weight. In addition, he received prescriptions for blood pressure and diabetes medications. Neither the nurse nor the RDN asked Jeff for his input regarding what changes he was willing to make.

Jeff found it difficult to comply with all aspects of his care. In his work life, he had many meetings and ate out quite often. He found it hard to watch what he was eating. What's more, he often forgot to take his pills, and his busy job also kept him from going to the gym. When he finally went back to see his doctor, he had gained weight, his hemoglobin A1C had increased by 2%, and his blood pressure was still elevated.

Ana's Story

Ana is a hair stylist who has been feeling very tired lately. She does not have health insurance. When she found out that a health fair in town was offering health screenings, she decided to go. At the health fair, she learned her blood glucose was elevated and she most likely has diabetes. Ana decided to see a doctor at a federally qualified health center close to her work. Since the clinic offered sliding-scale fees for office visits and medications, Ana was able to fit her care into her budget. At her first appointment, the doctor asked her the reason for her visit and what she was hoping to get out of the visit. Ana explained the results of her screening and that she wanted to learn more about diabetes, especially how to manage it. After confirming a diabetes diagnosis, the doctor explained to Ana that her hemoglobin A1C was 10%, what that number actually represented, and how medication would help her control her diabetes. He also explained that lifestyle changes would be very helpful and asked whether she would be willing to meet with an RDN for nutrition counseling. Ana agreed to schedule an appointment with the RDN, Marissa.

During their first meeting, Marissa started the appointment by asking Ana what her biggest concern was. Ana explained that she mainly was concerned with her new diagnosis of diabetes and that she did not want to go down the path that her mother and grandmother had followed. She was also concerned with the financial burden that diabetes may bring. Marissa addressed these concerns, explaining that diabetes care has changed a lot since her mom and grandmother were diagnosed. She also offered a referral to the social worker who worked at the clinic to assist with the financial concerns. Then Marissa continued the appointment by inquiring what Ana already knew about diabetes and how to manage it and what area(s) of self-care she wanted to address based on her current situation. As she found out more about Ana, Marissa offered some strategies Ana could choose that might fit into her lifestyle. With guidance from Marissa (who mainly asked open-ended questions), Ana chose a goal she believed to be a realistic starting point. She decided she would incorporate walking into her daily routine, and she and Marissa explored ideas for how she would accomplish this. Marissa reinforced how physical activity can positively affect Ana's blood glucose and overall health. Marissa also asked Ana whether she would like more resources to look over. Based on Ana's preferences, Marissa gave her a list of helpful websites and books. Marissa also provided information to Ana about low-cost and free community resources. Marissa offered to call Ana once a week to discuss the goal and assist with any questions she had.

Ana joined a weight-loss group and started walking most days of the week. Follow-up with Marissa and reading books about diabetes helped Ana to also change her cooking style and start eating smaller portions. By the time she returned 3 months later to see her doctor, Ana had lost weight, and her hemoglobin A1C had decreased to 7.8%. Plus, Ana reported that she had a lot more energy.

Comparing Ana's and Jeff's Stories

What is the difference between Ana's story and Jeff's? Is Ana more motivated than Jeff? Or is something else at work here?

Let's look first at Jeff's situation. The fact that he went to a renowned clinic where he received care from a group of medical experts did not improve his outcome. From the description of the encounter, it seems like Jeff did not have much of a role in developing the plan that he was responsible for implementing. The clinic he visited followed the "traditional" model of care, in which the health care professional is the authority responsible for the diagnosis and treatment as well as for the outcomes. In this model, patient education is generally prescriptive rather than collaborative. The health care professionals tell the patient what to do and set the goals for the patient. In Jeff's case, he was told that he had to change his diet, start to exercise, and lose weight. Nobody asked him what he wanted to do or how he wanted to approach his care. The health care team did not take his busy lifestyle into consideration. Their assumption was that Jeff was obligated to follow their advice and that he would figure out a way to integrate their suggestions into his lifestyle. Since Jeff did not follow the recommendations the experts gave him, he was labeled "noncompliant."

How about Ana? She went to a federally qualified health center—not the prestigious facility visited by Jeff. However, she succeeded in taking charge of her health outcomes. From the first interaction with a health care professional, she was asked the reason for her visit and what she was hoping to get out of it. The physician asked for Ana's agenda and did not impose his own. The RDN, Marissa, also asked Ana what she wanted to change and what she could reasonably achieve. Ana was part of the team. She worked *with* her health care providers instead of just following their directions. She set her own goals, and Marissa guided her to additional resources and information for managing diabetes. Marissa also helped Ana identify community-based support to help her in the future. What really makes the difference is listening to patients and involving them in their care.

As Jeff's and Ana's stories demonstrate, your work with patients will be more effective when you make sure that their self-management plans fit their specific goals and take into consideration their particular lifestyle and culture (for more details about cultural issues, refer to Chapter 10). Patients, not health care providers, should set the goals. When patients choose their own goals, they will be more apt to stick with them and do the work needed to achieve them. The goals will also fit their lifestyles better, because patients know what works and does not work for them.

To help our patients, it is important that we learn to work *with* our patients. One way of working with our patients is to use the empowerment approach.

The Empowerment Approach

Patient empowerment is one approach that can help patients identify the behavior they want to change and gives the RDN the opportunity to support them in this change. The empowerment approach is not just another tool we pull out of our kit when we are trying to help our patients to be more motivated and engaged. Instead, the purpose of patient empowerment, according to Funnell and colleagues, is to "help our patients recognize and develop the inherent capacity to be responsible for their own lives."[4] Patients are responsible for the majority of their own care. That is the reason that the patients are the final decision makers. The goal of the empowerment approach is to help patients take care of their chronic disease in a way that fits into their lives and their disease instead of expecting them to change their lives to meet the needs of their disease. The empowerment approach is a patient-centric approach; the patient is the center of the behavior change process. That is, the patient is the one who has to make the changes related to self-care and therefore must identify changes that he or she is willing to make. The patient needs to have the internal motivation for these changes to happen. *Goal setting with* the patient helps him or her learn how to make self-selected behavior changes, which in the long run will make the patient an "expert" in behavior change.[2,4,5,6]

In the traditional care model, the provider is "in charge" of the treatment decisions and ultimately responsible for the outcomes of the patient. A patient who does not follow the treatment recommendations is labeled as "noncompliant." The definition for *compliance* or *adherence* is "obedience"—obedience in following the rules established by the health care provider.[6] That is no longer true in the patient-centered care model; patients are in charge of making the decisions of what treatment options they want to follow and which they don't want to follow and therefore are responsible for the outcomes. Many of us health care providers are frustrated because we feel the patient should be following our recommendations; we have not yet made the shift to patient-centered care. Patient empowerment is not another method to improve patients' compliance or adherence.[6] Empowerment is collaboration between the patient and health care provider, where the patient is in charge of deciding what he or she wants to change and the RDN is there to support and assist the patient in making those changes.

To highlight the difference the empowerment approach can make, let's go back to Ana. Let's say that Ana is interested in having a piece of cake for her birthday. She asks Marissa if she can have the cake. There are several different answers that Marissa can give to Ana.

- Example 1: Marissa answers, "No, you can never have a piece of cake. You have diabetes!" Many of you know that this answer is wrong. We know that people with diabetes can eat cake, and it is not up to us to make that decision for them.
- Example 2: Marissa says, "Yes, but you can only have a small piece and you need to be careful." Is that the best answer? No, it is not, and let's explore the reason why this answer is not correct, either.

In Example 1, Ana eats the cake but feels guilty and is labeled as noncompliant and nonadherent because she is not following the recommendations of her RDN. She checks her blood sugar 2 hours after she eats the cake and the number is 289 mg/dL. In Example 2, Ana eats the cake and enjoys it. She checks her blood sugar 2 hours after she eats the cake and the result shows a blood sugar of 289 mg/dL. The blood glucose result or outcome is the same in both cases, but in Example 1 Ana is labeled as noncompliant and nonadherent because she did not follow the recommendations, while in Example 2 she is labeled compliant and adherent but her blood sugar was still elevated. In the empowerment approach, Marissa would actually tell Ana to make it into an experiment and check her blood sugar 2 hours after she eats the cake and then ask herself, "Was this the right decision for me today?" This approach allows patients to reflect on their own responses and lets them make different decisions based on the results that they are hoping to obtain.[6]

Implementing the Empowerment Approach

Empowerment is a philosophy in which the patient and the health care provider have their own roles.[2] You will want to clarify these roles during your first encounter with a patient. From the start of care, empowered patients play an active role. They give you feedback regarding what works and what does not work, and they tell you what their biggest concerns are. You are available to help and assist patients in the process. You partner with patients to help them choose goals and create action plans, and you help identify barriers to change as well as strategies to overcome them. You also collaborate with patients by providing care recommendations, expert advice, and support, maintaining a nonjudgmental attitude. In other words, you, as the health care provider, establish a partnership with the patient that is based on trust, respect, and acceptance. The patient has an opportunity to talk about his or her experience without feeling a need to shape the story to avoid disapproval or convince you that he or she made a "good choice." As the provider, you need to listen to the patient and find out what the patient needs to better manage his or her chronic disease.[6,7] As Funnell and colleagues stated, "Professionals need to give up feeling responsible *for* their patients and become responsible *to* them."[2]

Providing Information

In the traditional approach, clinicians provide education based on what *they* believe the patient needs to know. The provider assumes that the patient will change just by having the right information. The provider believes that change will occur if the patient understands how the body is supposed to work and what lifestyle changes need to be made to improve his or her health. The reality looks very different. Nobody has lost weight or changed eating habits simply by learning how the gut works and how food gets absorbed. Change does not happen just by increasing knowledge![8] Patients do want to learn, but they only want to learn what they feel is important to their life and their concerns right now. The education that an RDN provides is helpful, but the way the education is provided to the patient is what will make the difference.[2,6,7]

Patient education in the empowerment approach *does* include providing information, but only the information that the patient needs to know. The patient asks questions, and you provide the education that responds to these questions. You base education on the needs of the particular patient and do not provide instructions simply as part of "standard" care. You may consider starting the conversation by asking, "What would you like to know about high cholesterol or how elevated cholesterol affects your health?" The patient has a choice in deciding what information he or she needs to know in order to make better decisions related to his or her health. Of course, in some cases, a patient may not be sure what to ask; in such instances, you may offer some suggestions of topics that may be appropriate to discuss based on where the patient is currently in his or her disease process. Patients are also able to set the agenda to make sure their concerns and needs are being addressed. This approach can also be used in the classroom setting with group classes. Research supports that patients learn best when given the opportunity to ask questions.[2]

Besides knowledge, the patient also needs to learn how to make behavior changes and obtain ongoing support. The conversation will assist the patient in identifying what worked in the past and what did not work. It is also important to let patients identify which behavior they want and are willing to change. The RDN can assist patients in identifying past successes. In the empowerment approach, aspects of the chronic disease such as diet, monitoring, and medication are presented as tools that the patient can use to care for himself or herself, rather than as behaviors that the patient has to change.

In Ana's case, she learned about diabetes, her treatment options, and strategies. The education, however, was based on what she needed to know right now—not what might benefit her in 10 years. She did not learn about every medication on the market for diabetes. She learned only about the specific medication that she was going to take and how it would affect her daily life. Her education also focused on the lifestyle changes that she was able to make at this point in time. Because Ana could use the information right away, she knew what to expect and could better determine whether the medication was really making a difference in her diabetes as well as what impact the exercise had on her blood glucose. Giving patients the tools to be proactive is the main goal of the empowerment approach. Ana got the tools she needed to start taking care of her diabetes based on her current needs, desires, and cultural background. She also received access to resources so she could continue exploring other possible approaches. Finally, yet most importantly, Ana and her RDN worked together to create a goal and a plan.

Another part that is important but very often forgotten during a patient interaction is discussing and identifying psychosocial issues that the patient may have. Research shows that patients who have psychosocial issues may use health services more and also show lower levels of self-management behavior.[8,9]

Goal Setting

Goal setting is a very important part of the empowerment approach. The goal is a guide that helps each patient make lifestyle changes. These lifestyle changes eventually help patients improve their overall health and personal well-being.

For patients to be able to achieve mastery over their chronic disease and improve their quality of life, they have to learn to have self-confidence in the decisions they are making, to accept their disease and become experts in their body and the disease as it is related to their body. This, as a result, will provide them with emotional and physical well-being and make them behavior-change experts. In summary, patients have to become more self-directed and autonomous decision makers.[2] If our underlying purpose is to get patients to follow treatment recommendations—that is, to make them more "compliant"—then we are not using the empowerment approach.

Specific vs Overarching Goals

Most people are not able to change their behavior in 1 day. Lasting behavior change takes time and a lot of effort. Often, patients need help breaking down a large challenge into more manageable pieces that are easier to accomplish. You can play a crucial role in this process by assisting the person who has one or more chronic conditions to set realistic goals that he or she can achieve in a short period. We all have patients who would love to reach the stars and feel they need to set very ambitious goals. When working with such patients, our work is to help them understand the distinction between an overarching goal or outcome, on the one hand, and specific and achievable action steps over a short period, on the other.

How to Set Goals

Some patients may have a hard time identifying what they would like to work on. In these cases, you may want to help them identify something they previously tried and had success with. Is there anything that they would like to continue working on? Are there barriers they have identified that got in their way? What did they do to overcome them? Identifying barriers and having a plan in place to handle them is another important part of the goal-setting process.

The goal-setting process in the empowerment approach consists of five steps that help patients identify the information they need to develop and reach their health and lifestyle-related goals.[2,5] Box 3.1 (page 46) outlines these steps, along with questions you might use when working with patients.[2]

The first step of the process described in Box 3.1 ("Explore the problem or issue") provides the patient with the opportunity to define the problem. This initial step usually does not receive as much attention as it should, especially since it is not easy and many of us are tempted to go directly to the goal. Remember, a patient is only interested in changing something that he or she perceives as a problem. A patient who does not view smoking as a problem will not quit smoking; a patient who does not view obesity as a problem will not engage in weight loss. Many patients may not be aware of the problem that is getting in their way. Working through this first step will assist them in identifying what is not working for them right now. You can start the conversation by asking the patient, "What is your greatest concern? What is the hardest thing about caring for your chronic disease?"[2] Use open-ended questions and active listening to explore what is happening with the patient. The purpose of these questions is to focus the discussion on the patient's concerns about living with and caring for his or her chronic disease. Clinicians and patients often have different priorities about the most important issues related to a specific chronic disease. Patients are more   likely to make changes that will solve problems that are personally meaningful and relevant to them.

Box 3.1: Five steps for setting goals

Step 1: Explore the problem or issue (past)

- "What is the hardest thing about caring for your health condition?"

- "Please tell me more about that."

- "Are there some specific examples you can give me?"

Step 2: Clarify feelings and meaning (present)

- "What are your thoughts about this?"

- "Are you feeling (insert feeling) because (insert meaning)?"

Step 3: Develop a plan (future)

- "What do you want?"

- "How would this situation have to change for you to feel better about it?"

- "Where would you like to be regarding this situation in (specific time, eg, 1 month, 3 months, 1 year)?"

- "What are your options?"

- "What are barriers for you?"

- "Who could help you?"

- "What are the costs and benefits for each of your choices?"

- "What would happen if you do not do anything about it?"

- "How important is it, on a scale of 1 to 10, for you to do something about this?"

- "Let's develop a plan."

Step 4: Commit to action (future)

- "Are you willing to do what you need to do to solve this problem?"

- "What are some steps you could take?"

- "What are you going to do?"

- "When are you going to do it?"

- "How will you know if you have succeeded?"

- "What is one thing you will do when you leave here today?"

Step 5: Experience and evaluate the plan (future)

- "How did it go?"

- "What did you learn?"

- "What barriers did you encounter?"

- "What, if anything, would you do differently next time?"

- "What will you do when you leave here today?"

Adapted from Funnell MM, Anderson RM. Empowerment and self-management of diabetes. *Clin Diabetes*. 2004;22:123-127. Copyright 2004 American Diabetes Association. Reproduced by permission of the American Diabetes Association.

There is a saying related to active listening: "The word *silent* uses the same letters as *listen*." We need to be silent to hear the story our patients are sharing with us. To elicit the story, start with simple requests. Box 3.2 shows some examples.

Use care when using the word *why* to begin an open-ended question, especially if the question could sound judgmental. "Why?" can cause people to think you are blaming or scolding them, as in "Why did you eat so many snacks this week?" On the other hand, a well-phrased "why" question could help you and your patient understand better what is happening. An example is, "Why do you think it is so difficult to make time to walk after work?"

Box 3.2: Examples of open-ended questions

Open-ended question words	Example
Tell me more	Tell me how you feel about having this condition.
What	What is the most difficult thing about changing your eating habits?
	What is the hardest thing about having heart disease?
How	How do you feel when your blood pressure is elevated most of the time?

Avoid closed-ended questions like, "Did you take your insulin as directed this week?" This type of question puts the patient in a passive role where only a simple "yes" or "no" is required, and then the ball is back in your court. Ask instead, "How did you use your insulin this week?" and then sit back and listen!

In step two of Box 3.1 (page 46) "Clarify feelings and meaning", you work with the patient to explore his or her feelings, thoughts, and beliefs that may obstruct or help with goal achievement. Questions that you may consider asking include "How does the situation you just described make you feel? How will you feel if things change or do not change?" Patients seldom make and sustain changes in situations unless they care about solving the problem or improving the situation. Feelings are not problems that we are trying to solve. Emotions need to be explored, expressed, experienced, and accepted by the patient. The role of the RDN is to be thoughtful, compassionate, and an empathetic listener.[2]

The third step in Box 3.1 (page 46), "Develop a plan," will help the patient develop a long-term goal. He or she needs to identify what will work and what will not. Knowing the barriers to success is critical. In addition to discussing potential barriers, you can help the patient identify experiences or support that will help with goal achievement.[2]

Sometimes we feel our patients just do not have the willpower to change. Willpower is a reflection of two components: how important a goal is to the patient and how confident the patient is about accomplishing it. Working together will ensure the plan is important to the patient, giving him or her the "will," as well as the confidence to achieve it, giving him or her the "power." The RDN can help the patient increase his or her willpower by working on a problem that is meaningful and important to the patient.

In the fourth step of Box 3.1 (page 47) ("Commit to action"), the patient is ready to commit to a goal. During this step, you can help the patient be very specific and realistic, so the patient has a clear idea of what he or she wants to accomplish. Imagine a patient does not currently walk as far as the mailbox. If she sets a goal of walking 45 minutes a day, 7 days a week, she is being very specific but not realistic! Your role is to guide the patient toward what will work for him or her. (See Chapter 6 for more information on helping patients set goals that have a high probability of success.)

The final step from Box 3.1 (page 48) ("Experience and evaluate the plan") provides patients the opportunity to evaluate their efforts and identify what they learned in the process. Helping patients view this process as a behavioral experiment eliminates the concept of success and failure. Instead, all efforts are viewed as opportunities to learn more about the true nature of the problem, related feelings, barriers, and effective strategies. The role of the RDN is to provide information, collaborate during the goal-setting process, and offer support for patients' efforts.

Help your patients keep things in perspective during this last step. Some patients are not able to achieve the goals they chose and subsequently feel they have failed. How can we help patients in these circumstances? The purpose of this last step is to help the patient explore and learn from the experience. You can ask: How did it go? What did you learn from this experience? What would you change for next week? Whether the effort is successful or not, learning can still occur. In fact, some of our best lessons come from experiments that did not accomplish what we had planned. The fundamentals of empowerment and chronic disease are built on trial and error. This is a learning phase, helping the patient gain knowledge and confidence in how to make choices that are working for him or her.

People working on goals may be encouraged by Thomas Edison's attitude during his quest to invent the electric light: "I have not failed. I've just found 10,000 ways that won't work." More details on goal setting will be discussed in Chapter 6.

Practice Exercises

Exercise 1

As you work with patients this week, consider starting some of the sessions with open-ended questions, such as the questions listed in the first step of Box 3.1.

Exercise 2

Consider your own life and explore a concern you have by asking yourself open-ended questions. (Example: I am not making time to be physically active, even though I know it is good for my physical and mental health. What is the hardest part about being active? What am I willing to do to be more active?) Write down what you would like to accomplish.

References

1. Rubin RR, Anderson RM, Funnell MM. Collaborative diabetes care. *Pract Diabetol.* 2002;21:29-32.

2. Funnell MM, Anderson RM. Empowerment and self-management of diabetes. *Clin Diabetes.* 2004;22:123-127.

3. Glasgow RE, Anderson RM. In diabetes care, moving from compliance to adherence is not enough: something entirely different is needed [letter]. *Diabetes Care.* 1999;22:2090-2092.

4. Funnell MM, Anderson RM, Arnold MS, et al. Empowerment: an idea whose time has come in diabetes education. *Diabetes Educ.* 1991;17:37-41.

5. Anderson RM, Funnell MM, Barr PA, Dedrick RF, Davis WK. Learning to empower patients. *Diabetes Care.* 1991;14:584-590.

6. Anderson RM, Funnell MM. Ten things patient empowerment is not. *Treatment Strategies Diabetes.* 2010:2(1):185-192. http://viewer.zmags.com/publication /ad06b13c#/ad06b13c/184. Accessed May 13, 2015.

7. Anderson RM, Funnell MM. Patient empowerment: myths and misconceptions. *Patient Education and Counseling.* 2010;79:277-282.

8. Marrero DG, Ard J, Delamater AM, et al. Twenty-first century behavioral medicine: a context for empowering clinicians and patients with diabetes. *Diabetes Care.* 2013;36:463-470. http://care.diabetesjournals.org /content/36/2/463.full.pdf. Accessed May 15, 2015.

9. Peyrot M, Rubin RR. Behavioral and psychosocial interventions in diabetes. *Diabetes Care.* 2007;30:2433-2440. http://care.diabetesjournals.org/content/30/10/2433.full .pdf. Accessed May 15, 2015.

Chapter 4:
Are Your Patients
Ready to Change?

To work on a specific goal with a patient (especially a patient who was referred by another health care professional), you first determine how ready the person is to work on the goal. As we mentioned in Chapter 3, using open-ended questions as part of the empowerment approach is a key technique when it comes to goal setting. This communication method may be tied in with two other approaches: the transtheoretical model, also known as the stages of change model, and motivational interviewing. While the transtheoretical model and motivational interviewing are two distinctive methods, they are both patient focused and can help you identify the priorities of a patient and move the patient toward effective goal setting and accomplishment. This chapter will explore the stages of change model. See Chapter 5 for discussion of motivational interviewing.

Transtheoretical Model

Clinicians use the transtheoretical (stages of change) model to identify how ready a person is to initiate a particular behavior change. In the late 1970s and early 1980s, James Prochaska and Carlo DiClemente at the University of Rhode Island developed this model based on studies of how smokers were able to give up their habits. The idea behind their work is that behavior change does not happen in one step. Rather, most people have the tendency to progress through multiple stages on their way to a successful change. According to this model, a person can be "staged" based on his or her interest in and readiness to make a change.[1] Understanding a particular patient's stage or level of change helps you determine how to approach the person regarding a specific issue.

The stages of change are as follows[2]:

- Precontemplation—The person is not ready to make a change. He or she does not see that his or her behavior is a problem.
- Contemplation—The person is considering making a change but not right away. He or she knows the behavior is a problem but is not ready to make a change yet.
- Preparation—The person is getting ready to make a change soon.
- Action—The person has already taken steps toward making a change. Generally, only about 15% of people you initially meet with will be in the action stage.
- Maintenance—The person made a change and has been successfully working on it for at least the past 6 months.
- Relapse—The person has returned to the old behavior.
- Termination—The changed behavior has become a habit, and the person is absolutely certain that relapse will not occur.

The Significance of Staging

Remember Bob from Chapter 1? His doctor had told him that it would be a good idea to work with an RDN on weight loss and learning how to eat healthfully. In their initial session, the RDN followed her own agenda and made recommendations for Bob without assessing his readiness to change. The session was counterproductive. Bob did not follow her advice or return for another visit. Imagine how the outcome might have been different if the RDN had used the stages of change model. She would have recognized that Bob seemed to be in the precontemplation stage. He was not ready to hear her advice and, frankly, didn't see how his behavior was problematic.

Sometimes patients may not be ready to take action on a particular goal, especially if someone else is trying to set the goal for them. Resist the urge to use your expertise to "fix" such patients by telling them what to do. Instead, ask open-ended questions and listen carefully to your patients' answers to find out where they are and how they feel about a particular behavior change, as well as what they want to do. As you listen, determine where each patient fits in the stages of change model. Remember, when patients determine what goal they are willing to set, they are typically ready to work on this behavior. You will find that letting the patient set his or her own goals is the best approach, as it allows both the patient and you to have a positive and productive interaction.

In this chapter, we discuss how to identify the stage a person is in, and we suggest ways to approach a patient in each stage. When you start counseling a patient, your work will focus on helping this person progress from one stage to another, until he or she reaches the action phase. Later, when patients start making progress, you will employ strategies to help prevent relapse or moving back to earlier stages and old habits. As "change agents," we need to remember that change is not a straight line. In fact, people often move back and forth through various stages of readiness before they begin to take action. It's human nature!

Moving Through the Stages of Change: Jane's Story (Part 1)

Now let's meet Jane, a busy woman who is at risk for developing diabetes. Her physician referred her to an RDN, Kate, for weight-loss advice and support. At Jane's first appointment, Kate starts with an open-ended question: "How important is it for you to lose weight?" Jane's answer helps Kate to "stage" her and plan an approach for going forward with Jane.

Precontemplation

The following are some signs a person is in the precontemplation stage:

- The patient denies having a problem.
- The patient makes excuses (the "yes, but" syndrome).
- The patient blames others for his or her problems.

Jane, for example, may say she is too busy to prepare healthful food or it costs too much. She may even blame her husband for bringing the "wrong" foods into the house.

Precontemplation is the stage of resistance or reluctance, when patients may not be well informed about the benefits of a particular behavior change. You may see a need to educate them. However, to demonstrate to your patients that *they* are in charge of changing personal behavior, always ask them for permission before providing additional information.

Patients may have tried to make changes in the past but did not achieve success. They may think that a particular change is just not possible, despite knowing how important it may be. In these situations, you can help them overcome their lack of confidence regarding the issue. See Box 4.1 for additional counseling tips for the precontemplation stage.

Box 4.1: Counseling tips for the precontemplation stage

Acknowledge that your patient is not ready to make changes like losing weight or changing his or her diet. Accept that the patient may also not view a behavior change goal as important right now.

Affirm that the decision of what to do or not to do is entirely up to the patient.

Encourage the patient to consider the positive aspects of making a change.

Discuss what the patient thinks he or she *is* willing to change.

After they talk, Kate understands that Jane may not be ready to make any diet changes right now, even though she came to the session to learn about healthful eating. Jane may have initially focused on diet changes because her conversation with her physician led her to believe that eating is what she needs to change. Healthful eating may not really be her personal concern, or it may be an area that she has a low level of confidence in addressing. However, she states that she is willing to start taking walks in the evening.

Remember that a patient in the precontemplation stage in one area may be ready to make a change in another area, or even within different components of an area. For example, a patient who generally skips breakfast may be ready to start eating breakfast. However, expanding the goal to include carb counting or limiting fats at breakfast may be too overwhelming at the moment. Your job is to help the patient figure out (in great detail)exactly what he or she is ready to do and what barriers may get in the way.

What generally *doesn't* work for people in the precontemplation stage (or at any stage, for that matter) are threats of negative consequences. If you tell a person, "You are probably going to have a heart attack or stroke if you don't change your ways," he or she will usually ignore your statement. In fact, such threats often cause a person to "dig her heels in" and find more excuses *not* to change. If you are using threats with your patients, our advice to you is stop now! Threats just don't work.

Contemplation

Jane may recognize that her weight is a problem and may even want to do something about it. However, she has many hurdles she needs to overcome before she will be able to implement a change. She just needs to finish this big project at work and then she can make a plan and start working on it. Or, she just has to get through the holidays—everyone expects her to bake all of the holiday treats, and the kids and grandkids will be coming for an extended visit. A person in the contemplation stage generally isn't prepared to take action for at least another 6 months. See Box 4.2 for counseling tips for the contemplation stage.

Box 4.2: Counseling tips for the contemplation stage

People in the contemplation stage are fence sitters. We want to help them jump off the fence and start working on behavior changes that are meaningful to them. Some techniques you can employ are the same as those you would use for a person in the pre-contemplation stage:

- Acknowledge that the patient may not be ready to make changes in a particular behavior (or does not view that outcome as important right now).

- Affirm that the decision of what to do or not to do is entirely up to the patient.

- Encourage the patient to consider the positive aspects of making behavior changes.

- Work on the patient's ambivalence about the consequences of behavior change.

Patients in the contemplation stage are often ambivalent, or have mixed feelings, about the consequences of behavior change, and they may need to work through that phase before they are ready to change. You may want to ask patients in this stage to consider the negative and positive consequences of *not* changing, as well as the negative and positive consequences of making the change. (We will discuss ambivalence in greater detail in Chapter 5.)

Jane undertakes this exercise and identifies some of the benefits and consequences of making food changes to help with weight loss (see Box 4.3). Once Jane has completed her list, she and Kate can discuss the pros and cons. While discussing Jane's ambivalence, Kate begins to gain fresh insight into Jane's thoughts and feelings. More importantly, Kate helps Jane reflect on what these changes will or will not bring into her life. Jane now has a chance to evaluate what is more important for her. This conversation may help her tip the balance toward making a change. She may now be willing to discuss in more depth other things she can do to improve her health and which consequences matter to her.

Remember, if you are going to provide information to a patient, always ask for permission first. The patient needs to be ready to hear the information.

Box 4.3: Jane considers making a behavior change

Behavior	Advantages (pros)	Disadvantages (cons)
Not making diet changes	Can still eat all the foods I love. Don't have to plan meals. Can still eat fast food. No one tells me what to do.	May gain more weight. May end up developing diabetes like my sister.
Making diet changes	Will lose weight, feel better, fit into clothes I have outgrown. Will feel less embarrassed about body size, be healthier.	Have to deprive myself. Will be hungry all the time and can't eat foods I love. Need to find a different way to deal with stress.

Preparation

If Jane feels that weight loss is important and states she is ready to take action, she is probably in the preparation stage. In fact, she may have already started implementing some changes. At this stage, Kate focuses on helping Jane set an appropriate plan so she can succeed.

The patient in this stage will benefit from working on short-term goals and developing a plan for accomplishing them. Help your patients identify a measurable goal that is achievable within the next 1 to 2 weeks. You also want to help identify the barriers that could get in the way. See Box 4.4 for additional counseling tips for the preparation stage. By using these tips, you can develop a partnership with your patient. Keep in mind that the patient must be in complete control. You may have lots of great advice to offer, but the bottom line is that success depends on what the person does when he or she leaves your office. Your approach should focus on the person and take into account his or her readiness to make behavior changes.

Box 4.4: Counseling tips for the preparation stage

Help patients identify whom they can turn to for support, such as a spouse, a friend, or an actual support group.

Reinforce that patients have the skills to achieve their goals.

Affirm that small steps taken on a consistent basis result in success.

Action

By the action stage, you and your patients have built a successful partnership. They have set their goals and are achieving them. In this stage, you will help patients make adjustments so they can stay on track. What types of situations may make it difficult for individual patients to stick with their plans and reach their personal goals?

Jane has begun to include five to seven servings of fruit and vegetables in her diet each day. However, she is planning a vacation and will be eating out frequently. She is concerned it may be difficult to stick with her new eating habits and asks Kate for some assistance. Kate begins the discussion by asking her, "How are you planning to handle your meals while you are on vacation?" As Jane responds, Kate helps her identify possible solutions. Kate does *not* use her expertise as an RDN to create a list for Jane. After Jane has made her own list, Kate asks for permission to offer some additional tips. They also role-play some scenarios to help Jane prepare for vacation eating. Kate affirms the changes Jane has made thus far and reminds her that she has the skills to manage difficult situations.

People in the action phase are more successful if they have supportive relationships, especially at times when they are experiencing high levels of stress. Be sure to ask patients about their support systems. In addition, help them come up with healthful ways to handle temptations. For example, if nighttime snacking is a problem for Jane, taking a walk or phoning a friend may be healthful and helpful alternatives.

Maintenance

A patient in the maintenance stage has successfully adopted positive behavior changes and sustained those changes for at least 6 months. At this stage, follow-up is still important to prevent relapse. Your patients may even want to "plan for relapse" (ie, identify potential problem situations and put a plan for managing them in place). For example, Jane may be worried about the holiday meal at Thanksgiving. To plan for this potentially stressful time, she sets up appointments with Kate before and during the holidays. Kate also works with Jane to set up a Thanksgiving-specific plan to include more activity, eating healthful foods, and managing stress in positive ways. As you work with patients, ask them when they feel they may be most likely to relapse and plan strategies or visits around those situations.

During the maintenance stage, continue to help patients focus on the benefits of change. For example, Kate reminds Jane that she wants to make the meal plan change to help with weight loss so that she will feel better, prevent diabetes, and fit into her clothes.

Relapse (or Recycling)

Jane has been doing well making and sticking to behavior changes. In fact, she has lost weight and kept most of it off for over 2 years now. Her blood glucose, lipids, and blood pressure are under good control. She has not seen Kate in over 6 months. Life is good!

Kate worked with Jane in the maintenance phase to identify and plan for "trigger events." However, unexpected events like a death of a family member or friend, divorce, or job loss may lead Jane to deviate from her health plan. Even those patients who have incorporated a change into their lives for an extended period may go off track. For others, the change now seems to be second nature.

Patients may have feelings of disappointment, frustration, and failure if they relapse after having changes in place for a period of time, and they may not seek assistance. Affirm with patients that most people need more than one attempt to make a change, and life circumstances may cause them to get off track in the future.

Help your patients identify a course of action to take in case they unexpectedly relapse. The action plan may include increasing the frequency of visits with you or other health care providers.

Termination

When someone reaches the termination stage, the change has become second nature. Patients in this stage are not tempted to go back to the old behavior.

A person may reach the termination phase after being in the action stage for 6 months to 5 years. Generally, the new behavior has become a habit, like buckling up the seat belt when getting in the car or brushing teeth.

However, keep in mind that for some people, certain behaviors may never reach the termination stage. For example, Jane may always have to be aware of triggers that may cause a relapse. To help her, Kate encourages her to return once or twice a year for support and to continue working on the change.

Practice Exercises

Exercise 1

If you are meeting with patients who have goals "assigned" to them by their physician, ask them how ready they are to work on the goals. Identify their stage based on their response and use the strategies outlined in the chapter.

Exercise 2

Take a look at the accomplishment or change you wanted to achieve that you wrote down in Chapter 3. Now ask yourself how motivated you are to make that change. Identify what stage you are in currently. If you are not in the action phase, write down the benefits of making a change. Use Box 4.3 as an example.

References

1. Prochaska JO, DiClemente CC, Norcross JC. In search of how people change: applications to addictive behaviors. *Am Psychol*. 1992;47:1102-1114.

2. Prochaska JO. Decision making in the transtheoretical model of behavior change. *Med Decis Making*. 2008;28:845.

Chapter 5:
Moving Your Patients Toward Change: Motivational Interviewing

In Chapter 4, we reviewed the stages of change model and offered some suggestions for identifying how ready a person is to make a specific behavior change. This chapter focuses on another common technique used by practitioners: motivational interviewing (MI). This approach is based on a patient experiencing ambivalence and the health care provider helping the patient overcome this ambivalence and move toward change. Please note that to effectively use MI, training with ongoing coaching is recommended.[1]

The Origins of Motivational Interviewing

The clinical psychologist William R. Miller first described MI in 1983, and at that time the technique was mainly used to treat people who had a problem with alcohol.[2] He described motivation as being an interpersonal process that focuses on individual responsibility and internal desire to change. Later, Miller and Rollnick provided three different definitions for motivational interviewing: the definition used for the layperson, the definition used by the practitioner, and a technical definition. All three definitions include that MI is a person-centered, collaborative counseling style for strengthening the person's motivation and commitment to change by addressing the common problem of ambivalence to change.[3,4] MI strategies focus on guiding patients toward change but not on telling them what to do or attempting to "motivate" them. The practitioner is supportive of the choices the patients make, instead of telling them what is wrong with their choices, and practitioners also appeal to the internal motivation that all of us naturally have.[5]

Efficacy of Motivational Interviewing

The Academy of Nutrition and Dietetics Evidence Analysis Library examined four nutrition intervention studies that used RDNs trained in motivational interviewing. In all four studies, patients in the groups where MI was used achieved significantly better outcomes than the patients in groups where this strategy was not used. The improved outcomes included weight loss, better blood glucose control in people with diabetes, less consumption of fat, and adoption of low-fat methods to cook vegetables.[6-9] A literature review by Cummings and colleagues showed that MI is particularly useful with older adults.[10] According to the review, MI had a number of benefits for older adults with a variety of health issues, including becoming more physically active, improving their diets, lowering cholesterol and blood pressure, and improving blood glucose control. Based on these studies, the bottom line is that when MI is used with the appropriate patients by well-trained professionals who are skilled in MI, it works!

MI can help people overcome barriers to and build a personal case for change. Although motivational interviewing was initially used for treating addiction, it also can be used in the management of diseases that are directly or indirectly affected by the behavior of the person.

Basic Principles of Motivational Interviewing

Overview

MI involves several steps, along with the development of specific skills. It is a patient-centered method, in which the RDN or other counselor functions more as a guide than as a teacher. The purpose is to focus on one behavior, which is selected from a menu of choices generated by the patient, at a time.[11] When you use this technique, you ask strategic questions and then listen carefully to the patient's responses. This helps you determine whether the patient is willing to and interested in making a particular lifestyle change. One of the important premises of MI is this: *"If the change is important to the patient and the patient has the confidence to achieve the change, the patient will feel more ready to try to change and may be more successful at changing that particular behavior."*[3] If a person is not yet ready to make changes, "pushing" for a change can be counterproductive. Trying to make a patient institute a change before he or she is ready is like trying to get a 2-year-old to swallow a medication that tastes bad—the harder you try, the more the child resists. Most of us have some of that willful child in us; someone telling us what we should do can make us dig in our heels and do just the opposite. See Box 5.1 (page 74).

In the past, MI training focused mostly on the technique, in the *how* to do it, but was missing what the health care provider needs to be aware of when working with a patient. Miller and Rollnick defined these guiding principles as the *spirit of MI*. It is the mind-set and the heart-set that the health care provider needs to have in place for MI really to work.[3]

Box 5.1: The guiding principles of motivational interviewing

Guiding principle	Definition
Partnership	Building a partnership with the patient
Acceptance	Acceptance of where the patient is right now and what he or she is working on
Compassion	Compassion for who the patient is and what he or she is going through
Evocation	Bringing out the internal drive that is in the patient to change

As you work with MI, you first want to make sure that your patient is engaged in the conversation; otherwise, you are not going to get very far. The conversation needs to have a clear focus of what the patient wants to change. Once that is identified, you are able to evoke or elicit the patient's motivation to change. The patient first must decide whether he or she wants to change before he or she can decide how to change. These are the four key processes for MI to actually work:

- engaging—establishing a working relationship,
- focusing—developing and maintaining a specific direction of the conversation,
- evoking—eliciting the patient's motivations for change, and
- planning—developing both a commitment to change and a concrete plan.[3]

As we shall explore in the pages to follow, motivational interviewing helps patients identify ambivalence, which is a necessary first step toward moving them into action and changing behavior. Ambivalence can be defined as having mixed or contradictory ideas about something. Empathy is a key part of this collaborative approach; you will want to exhibit a willingness to understand the thoughts and feelings of your patients in order to help guide them through what is holding them back from or getting in the way of a self-selected change.

To most effectively help patients identify ambivalence, you will need to be comfortable with the four core communication skills used throughout MI, which are known as OARS: asking open-ended questions, affirming, reflecting, and summarizing. These communication techniques provide patients with a safe and accepting environment that helps them express their personal thoughts, feelings, and experiences. It's important to always remember that the patient determines the pace and the direction of the counseling session. Throughout the process, patients decide whether they want to make a change and what they want to change, and then they set their own goals. You are an adviser, asking questions to help the person identify an area of concern and develop a plan that he or she wants to accomplish and is confident about. You may also offer suggestions, after first asking the patient if he or she is open to hearing your ideas. The most important things to remember are to listen more, advise less, and ask open-ended questions.[2,3,11]

Ambivalence

Addressing ambivalence is the cornerstone of motivational interviewing. Most people who are interested in making a change have some feelings of ambivalence about making the change happen. Typically, if patients are experiencing feelings of ambivalence, they are a step closer to changing. They are actually thinking about making a change, but they are not sure if the energy that they have to invest is worth it. They are on the right track toward making a change, but on the other hand, patients who are ambivalent may never change because they cannot find enough reasons to change—they can get stuck.

Ambivalence is simultaneously wanting and not wanting something.[3] A person who experiences ambivalence will often perceive advantages and disadvantages in both maintaining a current behavior and changing to a new behavior. When you are working on ambivalence with a patient, you may want to use the technique we discussed in the "Contemplation" section of Jane's story in Chapter 4—ask the patient to consider the negative and positive consequences of *not* changing as well as the negative and positive consequences of making the change. This way, the patient has a chance of seeing the pros and cons of making or not making a change. With the patient, you can also spend some time looking at perceived barriers to change and guide him or her toward naming solutions to barriers.[12]

Box 5.2 is an example of a decisional balance tool that you may use to help someone having difficulty committing to a course of action to explore advantages and disadvantages of change versus status quo. (We have already seen how this tool can be used in the case study of Jane in Box 4.3 on page 63.) While decisional balance tools may be helpful, they are not an integral part of MI. They may allow some patients to more clearly see what is influencing their decisions regarding change, but they are not necessary for every patient.[11]

Box 5.2: Decisional balance tool for exploring ambivalence

Behavior	Advanatages (pros)	Disadvantages (cons)
Not making the behavior change	What do you like about your current behaviors?	What don't you like about staying the same?
Making the behavior change	What good will happen as a result of making a change?	What don't you like about making change?

Motivational interviewing regards ambivalence as a part of the natural process of altering one's behavior, a phase that people have to go through before they can change. As we have noted in previous chapters, some RDNs feel that they need to lecture patients about the benefits of eating healthier food. These RDNs understandably want to share their wealth of knowledge. However, this approach often results in the patient becoming even more resistant to change. While the RDN is trying to "push" the patient into adopting a new behavior, the patient is instead affirming why he or she doesn't want to change.[12] For example, imagine a patient who is debating whether to avoid eating a bedtime snack 2 times a week. The RDN may be arguing in favor of the change and does not give the patient time to think through the pros and cons of making or not making the change. The natural reaction of the patient in this situation is to argue against the change because he or she feels pressured by the RDN. The patient will become resistant to change, and the opportunity has been lost! The patient, not the clinician, needs to be the one who identifies the benefits and the costs to making or not making the change.

Open-Ended Questions

We mentioned in Chapters 3 and 4 the importance of using open-ended questions to elicit discussions with your patients. In this section, we will explore in more detail how you can implement these questions when using MI techniques. Open-ended questions are a great conversation-starting tool to use in social settings, too![12]

An open-ended question is like an open door; it invites the person to think a bit more before responding and provides plenty of latitude for how to answer. The goal of open-ended questions is to obtain the patient's story. You need to be curious and try to understand the experience of the person and the meaning that the person attributes to that particular experience. This is quite different from the way many of us have been trained to gather information. We tend to follow a protocol or ask a series of specific questions to help "get the facts." We may even interrupt the patient.

In MI, the open-ended questions help you understand where people are coming from, their internal frame of reference. Understanding this better will allow you to strengthen the collaboration and find the direction the patient wishes to take. The open-ended questions also play a key role in evoking motivation and planning a course toward change.[3] For more information on open-ended questions, refer to Box 3.2 (page 49).

Affirmations

MI builds on the patient's own personal strengths, efforts, and resources. It is the patient who produces change, not the clinician. The role of the RDN is to monitor the desire and ability of the patient to make a change and help guide him or her, but it is the patient who will eventually have to make the change.

Affirmations can be a useful tool for the RDN. Affirmations are a simple way for the RDN to show the patient appreciation and understanding. This helps to build and maintain rapport. The RDN can affirm the patient by acknowledging his or her efforts to make changes, no matter how large or small. One way of using affirmation is self-affirmation. Ask the patient to describe his or her own strengths, past successes, and positive efforts. This gives patients the opportunity to hear themselves describe how they reached a goal in the past, and it will help them realize that they have the ability to tackle the new goal you are setting together. This approach can also be used as you explore with patients what has worked in the past and why.[3]

An affirmation and praise are not the same. The big difference is that in an affirmation, you communicate the "value" of the person and his or her behavior, while praise may be perceived as passing judgment on behavior. An example of an affirmation is, "Following your action plan helped you lose 10 pounds over the past 4 months." In contrast, an example of praise is, "Congratulations, I am so proud of you for losing 10 pounds."[12] Using the word *I* puts a parental undertone into the sentence. Also, we do not know if the patient is really excited about the weight loss. The person may have hoped for more and is very disappointed that he or she lost only this amount.

Reflective Listening

The reflective listening technique is an integral skill to develop when using the MI approach. Reflective listening, used correctly, is probably one of the most important communication skills, but it can be a difficult skill to master. This is because it requires the listener to totally drop his or her own agenda. The speaker becomes the center of attention and the listener makes no attempt to influence the speaker's perception or what he or she is saying. The speaker's report is accepted as given. The goal is to listen and strive to understand the meaning of what the speaker is saying.[3,12,14] To use this technique, listen carefully, and then, once the patient is finished speaking, repeat or restate what he or she just told you. Operationally, you, as the listener, are functioning as a mirror that is reflecting back what the speaker has said. Pose your response as a statement, not a question. A question requires an answer, while a reflection allows the patient to confirm or clarify and further explore what is happening and why.[3,12]

Reflective listening thus shows a patient you are listening and you understand what he or she is saying. The effective use of reflective listening also keeps the conversation moving forward, closer to goal setting and behavior change.[3] Reflective listening can feel unnatural at first, but as with most skills, it does get easier with practice. Just be careful not to overuse this approach. You do not want to sound like you are repeating every single thing your patient is saying. The following is an example of a script you might use:

> **Patient**: "It's just too hard. I don't want to change my diet."
>
> **RDN**: "You don't want to change your diet because you find it easier to keep it the same."

Alternately, you may rephrase what the patient just said:

> **Patient**: "I really want to start exercising again."
>
> **RDN**: "Sounds like you are ready to start exercising again."

You may want to reframe what the patient said to put a positive and encouraging spin on it:

> **Patient**: "I have tried so many times to lose weight, but I am never successful."
>
> **RDN**: "Your efforts say a lot about your perseverance and how important weight control is for you. Even though it has been difficult for you, you don't give up!"

Rolling with Resistance

Rolling with resistance is another skill that is widely used in MI. Directly challenging a patient about a lifestyle behavior is counterproductive because the confrontation typically results in the patient defending the current behavior. Instead, MI advocates the principle of "rolling with resistance." When you roll with resistance, you give recognition to the natural ambivalence that is part of being human. From this perspective, resistance is viewed as a normal process to be expected rather than as a threat to your authority or expertise. So, instead of meeting a patient's resistance head on, you acknowledge the resistance and step aside, figuratively speaking. When you acknowledge resistance, it tends to lose its intensity. If you align with the patient to address the issues together, the energy behind the resistance can sometimes be channeled into small steps toward change. However, this is not to imply that you can never disagree with a patient's viewpoint.[13]

Summaries

Summaries are a nice way to move from one topic to the next or to highlight some of the ambivalence that you have identified in the patient. You may also want to use a summary at the end of the appointment to recap the major points of discussion.[11] When you summarize, you generally start with a statement that describes what you and your patient talked about. After making this statement, you then list some of the key items you and your patient have just discussed. This is a point where you can also refer to any ambivalence that you and the patient noted. You then invite the patient to add anything to the summary that you may have missed. To end a summary while keeping the conversation moving forward, ask an open-ended question.[3]

Here is an example:

> **RDN:** You have brought up several issues that you are interested in exploring further. These include your diabetes not being under optimal control and your late-night eating habits; you enjoy food, but you mentioned that you are frustrated with not being able to lose any weight despite all the efforts you have made. We want to discuss all these issues, but which one would you like to focus on for today's appointment?

Providing Advice

With MI, you reserve your advice for the patient until late in the conversation. This last phase comes into play after the patient states what he or she wants to do. If you have concerns about the patient's thinking on the subject, ask for permission to share some thoughts with him or her. If the patient grants permission, you can then offer suggestions and share some of what you learned from those years of education and experience! But be careful— remember the patient's opinion is what matters most, not yours. Here are a few examples:

- Do you mind if we spend a few minutes talking about the effect of the different fats on your heart disease?
- What do you know about celiac disease? Would you be open to looking at some food items that you might find when you eat out, as discovering all of the wheat in restaurant food can be tricky?
- Are you interested in learning more about how you can adjust your insulin based on the carbohydrates you consume?

What to Do When a Patient Clams Up or Spouts Off

Sometimes it may seem like you just are not connecting with a patient. The patient may be quick to argue, ignore you, or answer, "Yes, but." When this happens, remember that communication is a two-way street. If you are feeling frustrated about your conversation with a patient, the patient is likely feeling the same way. Your conversation may be entering an area the patient is not ready to explore, or you may be giving advice when he or she is not ready to receive it.

The following are a few things to ask yourself in these situations:

- Do I really know how the patient feels about this topic? Ask the patient if he or she is interested in or ready to address the issue. The transtheoretical (stages of change) model may help you "stage" the person.
- Why is the patient feeling so strongly about this?
- Am I allowing the patient to control which issues we discuss, or am I being preemptive?
- Am I being a teacher and telling the patient what to do?
- Have I been listening more than talking?

Next, take steps to diffuse the situation:[12]

- Make sure you are using reflective listening.
- Empathize with the patient and normalize actions: "Most people make several attempts before they are able to lose weight."
- Disclose something about your own experiences, if appropriate: "I also used to be overweight. Even as a dietitian nutritionist with all the right knowledge, I had a difficult time making diet and physical activity changes." Keep any self-disclosure short and simple. The appointment is about your patient, not you.
- Get back to asking what the patient wants to talk about.
- Make certain the patient knows your goal is not to "make" him or her change. You are simply there to support what the person wants, which may or may not include behavior change.

Optimizing the Results of Motivational Interviewing

When coupled with other interventions, MI can be an even more powerful tool in patient behavior change. What else do we need to do to help our patients? Based on a systematic literature review and meta-analysis, Rubak and colleagues concluded that the time spent with the patient, the frequency of the visits, and the length of the visits were equally important in helping a patient make changes.[5] The following are some of the points to take away from this research:

- Meet with each patient several times, if possible. When MI was used in one encounter with patients, about 40% of them showed a positive effect. When the number of encounters was 5 or more, the number of patients making changes increased to 87%!

- Longer sessions may be more successful than shorter sessions, but brief encounters (eg, 15 minutes) are still useful—81% of subjects in sessions that were 60 minutes in length showed positive changes, and 64% showed a positive effect when sessions were briefer than 20 minutes.

- Follow-up is key. Among participants who were followed for at least 1 year, 81% showed improvement, whereas 36% showed positive effects when followed for 3 months.

- The impact of MI is closely related to the duration and number of encounters between the patient and the provider and less strongly associated with the education the patient received. Practitioners trained in MI make a difference in patient outcomes!

- Practice your listening skills with patients and family members. If you want a real challenge, try it out with a teenager who has been giving you grief!

James's Story

James is a 52-year-old male with hypertension who has two adult children. He recently saw his physician and received a referral to see Laura, the RDN who is part of the team to help James get better control of his blood pressure and to lose some weight.

> **Laura:** Thank you for coming in. I see that you recently saw Dr O'Connor and he wants us to work together. Is that correct?
>
> **James:** Yes, Dr O'Connor thinks I am not doing a good job with my health.
>
> **Laura:** I am looking here at your chart, and it looks like several of your blood pressure readings have been high, in the range for you to be considered hypertensive.
>
> **James:** Does that mean I have high blood pressure?
>
> **Laura:** Yes, high blood pressure is also called hypertension. A person is said to be hypertensive if his systolic (higher number) is at or greater than 140 or his diastolic (lower number) blood pressure is at or greater than 90. What do you make of that?
>
> **James:** I don't know; I don't feel like my blood pressure is high…

Laura: It's true, high blood pressure often goes unnoticed by many people because there are very few symptoms. Most people report feeling just fine! *(reflection—giving back, giving information, and validating the patient's experience)*

James: Yes, I do feel pretty good. But I guess I am not that surprised. I am a smoker and have put on a bit of weight over the years, and I know these things probably don't help. But I just can't seem to resist my smokes and snacks! *(ambivalence)*

Laura: You are pretty knowledgeable about the risks for high blood pressure!

James: Yes, but knowing what's bad for you and changing are two very different things.

Laura: Of the things you mentioned—smoking, your weight, and snacking—I wonder if you could tell me about which of these, if any, concerns you most. *(asking open-ended questions)*

James: Well, we hear so many bad things about smoking these days, and I have tried to quit at least five times, but nothing I've tried has ever worked, so I have just given up.

Laura: Tell me what concerns you about your smoking.

James: Well, my father smoked for over 40 years and died of a heart attack at the age of 60, which is only 8 years away! I guess I don't want to end up like him.

Laura: It sounds like there's a lot more life you want to live… *(reflection)*

James: Yes, I want to retire in a few years and my wife and I have plans to travel. And I notice that just going to the store tires me out… leaves me out of breath.

Laura: It sounds like it's important to you to be able to travel without feeling tired and breathless. *(reflection)*

James: It is, but like I said, I have tried so many times to quit without success. I have just about given up. *(ambivalence and resistance)*

Laura: When was the last time you tried quitting?

James: Oh, about 10 years ago, I guess—it's been a while. I tried the gum and just going cold turkey, but neither worked.

Laura: It has been a while! You know, there are many new things that have been developed in the past 10 years to help people quit, many of which you may not have tried. Would you like me to tell you about some of them?

James: Sure, why not!

Laura: Well, there is the nicotine patch; there is also medication, which helps as well. A couple of my patients have tried it and feel it really works. Also, studies show that people who get regular support when they first quit smoking are also more successful—quit lines work well and are easy to use, and some are free of charge.

James: Do you think that if I try one of these that it may help me to quit?

Laura: They certainly might. The question is how ready and motivated do you think you are to make a change now, let's say, on a scale from 0 to 10 (where 0 is not at all motivated and 10 is completely motivated)? *(assessing readiness and motivation for change)*

James: I would say about a 7 or 8. I would really like to quit for all the reasons I mentioned, even though I like to smoke. *(some ambivalence but starting to hear some change talk)*

Laura: That's pretty motivated! Now tell me, why are you at a 7 or 8 and not a 2 or 3?

James: Well, like I said, I really don't want to end up like my dad, who died really young. I am also looking forward to my retirement, and I know how much my wife is looking forward to traveling—I don't want to disappoint her!

Laura: It sounds like you want to be healthy enough to enjoy a long and happy retirement with your wife. *(reflection)*

James: Yes, exactly.

Laura: Now, sometimes wanting to change isn't enough to make it happen, like you mentioned earlier. So we like to ask people about how confident they feel in their ability to change. So, on the same scale from 0 to 10 (where 0 is not at all confident and 10 is very confident), if you decided to quit smoking now, how confident do you feel in your ability to quit? *(assessing self-efficacy)*

James: That one is trickier. As I said, I have tried to quit at least five times and without success. Though I have never tried the patch or the medications you mentioned, which might work. *(change talk)* I would say I am about a 4 or 5 on confidence; I hope I can, but I am not sure I can do it.

Laura: So you are moderately confident. What do you think it would take to get you to a higher number (that is, what would it take to boost your confidence)?

James: Um, I'm not sure. I know I have a hard time remembering to take pills (and I hate taking pills!), so maybe trying the patch would be more realistic for me because I would just have to stick it on and I could forget about it. And I guess I could get my wife to remind me to change it… I am sure she'd be happy to help.

Laura: So, knowing yourself, the patch sounds like a good place to start. And having your wife's support would certainly help! *(reflecting back and reinforcing plan)* When do you think you'd be ready to start the patch?

James: Well, I guess right away. Do I need a prescription?

Laura: Yes, and once you start, we can follow your progress to see how it's working. How does that sound?

James: That sounds good to me!

Practice Exercises

Exercise 1

Choose something that you have been thinking about changing—something that you are ambivalent about. Ask someone at work or at home to work with you. You will need to explain to your helper that you want him or her to help you through two scenarios.

> **Scenario 1:** The person who is helping you needs to tell you how much you need to make this change, how to do it, and the reason why. How did you respond? What feelings did you experience?

> **Scenario 2:** You do that again, but you ask the person who is helping you not to give you any advice; instead, the helper asks a series of questions and listens carefully and respectfully to what you have to say. Here are some examples of questions that the helper may want to ask: Why would you want to make this change? How might you go about it in order to succeed? What are the three best reasons for you to do it? How important is it for you to make this change, and why? Your helper listens to the answers and at the end provides a summary of what he or she heard. As with Scenario 1, how did you respond? What feelings did you experience?

Discuss with your helper what scenario worked best for you and how your helper felt about each scenario. This is a great example of the person-centered spirit and style of MI. What you just experienced yourself is the different dynamics of a conversation! So what do you think you will do? Will you actually change, or are you going to resist the change?

Exercise 2

Practice reflective listening with patients using the techniques listed in this chapter—repeating, paraphrasing, or offering a positive spin.

Exercise 3

Consider asking one or two patients if you can tape your sessions and listen to the tapes to see if you are using any of the techniques we discussed in this chapter.

References

1. Miller WR, Rollnick S. Ten things that motivational interviewing is not. *Behav Cognit Psychol*. 2009;37:129-140.

2. Miller WR. Motivational interviewing with problem drinkers. *Behav Psychother*. 1983;11:147-172.

3. Miller WR, Rollnick S. *Motivational Interviewing: Helping People Change. 3rd ed.* New York, NY: Guilford Press; 2013.

4. Miller WR, Rollnick S. *Motivational Interviewing: Preparing People to Change Addictive Behavior.* New York, NY: Guildford Press; 2002.

5. Rubak S, Sandbaek A, Lauritzen T, Christensen B. Motivational interviewing: a systematic review and meta-analysis. *Br J Gen Pract*. 2005;55:305-312.

6. Bowen D, Ehret C, Pedersen M, et al. Results of an adjunct dietary intervention program in the Women's Health Initiative. *J Am Diet Assoc*. 2002;102:1631-1637.

7. Resnicow K, Jackson A, Wang T, et al. A motivational interviewing intervention to increase fruit and vegetable intake through black churches: results of the Eat for Life Trial. *Am J Public Health*. 2001;91:1686-1692.

8. Smith DE, Heckemeyer CM, Kratt PP, Mason DA. Motivational interviewing to improve adherence to behavioral weight control program for older obese women with NIDDM. *Diabetes Care*. 1997;20:52-54.

9. West DS, DiLillo V, Bursac Z, Gore SA, Greene PG. Motivational interviewing improves weight loss in women with type 2 diabetes. *Diabetes Care*. 2007;30:1081-1087.

10. Cummings SM. Motivational interviewing to affect behavioral change in older adults. *Res Social Work Pract*. 2005;19:195-204.

11. American Association of Diabetes Educators. *The Art and Science of Self-Management Education: A Desk Reference for Health Care Professionals.* Chicago, IL: American Association of Diabetes Educators; 2006.

12.   Borrelli B. Using motivational interviewing to promote
       patient behavior change and enhance health. Medscape.
       http://www.esrdnetwork6.org/diamond/Missed%20
       Treatments/MT-14.pdf. Published July 28, 2006. Accessed
       June 28, 2015.

13.   VanWormer JJ, Boucher JL. Motivational interviewing and
       diet modification: a review of the evidence. *Diabetes Educ.*
       2004;30:404-414.

14.   Rollnick S, Mason P, Butler C. *Health Behavior Change:
       A Guide for Practitioners.* London, England: Churchill
       Livingstone; 2000.

Chapter 6:
Putting the WHAT
into Goal Setting

The reason most people never reach their goals is that they don't define them, or ever seriously consider them as believable or achievable. Winners can tell you where they are going, what they plan to do along the way, and who will be sharing the adventure with them.

—Denis Waitley

Most of our patients have heard advice from their health care professionals like lose weight, exercise more, cut down on saturated fat, reduce your salt intake, or get more fiber into your diet. Unfortunately, many of our patients do not know how to translate these broad goals into their everyday lives. As RDNs, we can help our patients quantify and develop action plans around outcomes like "eat less saturated fat" or "lose weight."

In previous chapters, we talked about letting patients set their own agendas—each patient should determine what he or she is interested in working on. Your next objective is to guide patients into action. Once they are ready to make a change and have identified where they would like to start, you will help them set achievable goals. One key to setting goals is *desire*—the goal has to be something the patient wants to do. The second key is *confidence*—the goal needs to be something the patient is fairly certain he or she can accomplish. The third key, which we will cover in this chapter, is how to help your patients set *very specific goals* or action plans. Finally, to succeed in achieving their goals, patients also need frequent follow-up.[1-4]

Fostering Confidence

If patients have desire and confidence, they should be able to successfully initiate health changes, with your guidance and support. Self-efficacy (or confidence) is one's ability to change and achieve healthier behaviors. Bodenheimer and colleagues showed that even patients who have a low income level and obtain their care through safety-net clinics were able to set and achieve goals as often as higher-income patients who were seen in private practices, as long as they wanted to change and believed it was possible for them to change.[5]

In Chapter 7, we will go into more detail about emotional health issues and other stressors that may prevent a person from having the desire and confidence to change. These obstacles can include high anxiety levels, depression, lack of money, family concerns, or competing time issues. For some patients, the first steps may be to identify any such concerns in their lives and to find out where to go for assistance. Until they take these steps, they cannot embark on lifestyle changes such as increasing physical activity, eating more healthfully, or ceasing tobacco use.

As we mentioned in Chapter 3, some patients may feel more confident if they view the goal as something they can try out, like an experiment. This way, if they do not achieve it, they may be less likely to perceive themselves as failures.

The WHAT System

As we have discussed in previous chapters, patients who are ready to change will be more successful if they set their own goals. Broad objectives are not enough. Goals must be specific and achievable, tailored to the individual's lifestyle and culture. To help your patients with goal setting, we created the WHAT system:

- *W* stands for *what* the patient will do, *when* he or she will do it, and *where* he or she will do it.
- *H* is for *how much* or *how many* and *how often*.
- *A* stands for *achievable* (and believable).
- *T* represents the *time frame* for accomplishing the goal.

The more precise the goal or action plan is, the easier it will be for the patient to incorporate it into his or her life. See Table 6.1 (page 100) for tips on refining initial goals so they are specific and achievable.

Table 6.1: Goal-setting tips

Original goal	Concerns	Techniques to improve goal	Possible new action step
Lose weight	Action is not specific	Identify action linked with weight loss that the patient wants to try.	I will walk 20 minutes after dinner every other day after dinner.
Walk more, eat less, drink more water, avoid sweets, eat more vegetables, lift weights, do yoga	Too many goals	Help the patient choose one or two specific goals to work on and track.	I will pack fresh veggies as part of lunch this work week. I will have salad with dinner three days this week.
Doctor said to avoid white flour and sugar	Goal does not identify what patient wants to do	Help the patient set a reasonable action plan. Communicate with the patient's doctor.	I will drink water or diet soda in place of regular soda once per day during the work week. I will buy whole grain bread to use in place of white bread for sandwiches.

Original goal	Concerns	Techniques to improve goal	Possible new action step
Eat less	Goal is too vague	Help the patient create a specific action plan.	I will drink only water after dinner (no snacks or calorie-containing liquids) 5 days this week (Sunday–Thursday).

Jane's Story (Part 2)

You met Jane and her RDN, Kate, in Chapter 4. Jane is interested in losing weight and is willing to make some diet changes to achieve that objective. How can Kate use WHAT to help her?

What, When, and Where?

Let's start with W—*what* will the patient do, *when* will she do it, and *where* will she do it? To start with goal setting, Kate asks for permission to advise Jane on potential meal plan changes that may help with weight loss. Jane settles on incorporating more fruits and vegetables in her eating plan—that action is the *what*.

Then Kate asks Jane *when* she wants to work on incorporating more fruits and vegetables. Jane decides to start with lunch. She often brings a lunch from home to work and frequently supplements it with vending machine items like chips and candy. She decides that she will bring some fruit and veggies to work as part of her lunch instead of purchasing items from the vending machine. In making this plan, Jane also answers *where*—she will work on her goal at her worksite.

How?

Now the questions to ask are *how much* or *how many* and *how often.* Jane decides that she will supplement her lunch with one piece of fruit and a small bag of raw veggies (thus answering, "How many?"). For *how often,* Jane says that she wants to do this every workday—that is, Monday through Friday.

Achievability

Next Kate helps Jane determine whether this goal is *achievable* for her. Does Jane *believe* that she will be able to pack fruit and raw vegetables for every lunch and not use the vending machines? To make it easier for her to avoid vending machine purchases, Jane said she will leave her cash at home. There is no ATM nearby, and she usually uses her credit or debit cards for other types of purchases. Plus, she knows that she would not feel comfortable asking her coworkers to loan her money for vending machine purchases. Jane also decides to stock up on different kinds of fruits and vegetables when she does her weekly shopping.

Time Frame

Now for the *time frame*: Typically, you will help patients set an action plan or goal that can be accomplished during the next 1 to 2 weeks and then have them follow up with you at the end of the time period. Sometimes people find they have problems achieving their goals, despite your best efforts to help them develop a WHAT plan. If that is the case, you will want to help the person revise the plan sooner instead of later. If the goal does not work, some people will throw up their hands and give up on the goal. If they know they are going to check in with someone regarding their goals, they are often less likely to totally dismiss their action plan. Understanding this, Kate sets up a follow-up visit for Jane in 2 weeks.

Putting WHAT into Action

Before the action plan is launched, Kate can verbally summarize the goal for Jane—to bring a piece of fruit and a bag of veggies for lunch from Monday through Friday for the next 2 weeks—and invite her to write it down, if she desires. If Jane seems hesitant to write out her goal, Kate could also offer to write it down for Jane. However, it can be empowering to patients if they write it out themselves. Once the goal is written, Kate shares with Jane that some people find it helpful to post the goal in a visible location and track their progress through keeping a log.

Next Kate takes the final step in setting the goal: She affirms Jane's confidence level in achieving her action plan. Kate asks Jane to use a 0-to-10 confidence scale to measure her certainty of whether or not she can accomplish her action plan (Figure 6.1, page 104). Zero means that she is absolutely sure she *cannot* meet her goal and 10 indicates that she is completely certain that she *will* do it. People who score 7 or higher on the confidence scale are most likely to succeed. If Jane does not score at least 7,

Kate will want to help her adjust her goal. Jane says the goal will be a big change for her, but she wants to make the change and she is fairly certain that she will be successful. She rates her confidence level as a 7.

Figure 6.1: Confidence scale

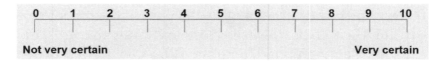

Following Up: Adjusting the Goal as Needed

At her follow-up visit, Jane shares her progress toward achieving her goal with Kate. Jane reports that she was not completely successful. The first week she brought the fruit and veggies every day, but she ate them on only 4 out of 5 days. On the fifth day, she went out to lunch. The following week, she brought and ate the fruit and vegetables on 3 days, and she did not have time to prepare veggies for the fourth and fifth days. On those days, she brought money to work to purchase items from the vending machine.

Jane's account illustrates why follow-up is so critical. Jane was successful some of the time. The follow-up appointment is an opportunity for Jane and Kate to explore what Jane learned from the experiment and redefine the goal as needed. Kate asks, "What got in the way of you achieving your action plan?" Jane replies that sometimes she is too busy and does not have time to prepare the lunch as planned. Kate also asks Jane what she learned about herself. Jane replies that eating with friends is very important and that she felt that the current goal did not provide the flexibility in doing that. Kate then asks Jane how she would like to revise her goal so that she can accommodate eating out at lunch. Jane says perhaps 3 to 4 days a week of bringing the fruit and veggies for lunch would be more realistic. Kate also asks about Jane "not having time" to prepare vegetables: "Is there something that you would do differently so that you make certain you have veggies ready and available for lunch?"

In situations like Jane's, you may find that patients don't seem to have a ready solution in mind. To help Jane problem solve, Kate uses a technique known as "brainstorming." The brainstorming guidelines listed in Box 6.1 (page 106) are based on those used in the Stanford Chronic Disease Self-Management Program.[6]

In response to Jane's comment that she ran out of time to prepare vegetables, Kate asks her if she would like to think of ways to make sure she has veggies ready for her lunch. Jane lists some ideas, such as shopping more often, buying vegetables that are already cut up, or leaving a big bag in the office refrigerator so she doesn't have to prepare them every day. Kate asks for permission to add other ideas to her list, and then suggests that Jane buy frozen or canned vegetables, keep some frozen or canned vegetables at work, make casseroles that have extra vegetables in them to take to work, or consider purchasing some dried vegetables.

Next Kate asks Jane to consider what is on the list and identify one possible solution she would like to try over the next week. Jane looks the list over and states she hadn't really thought about keeping frozen vegetables at work. She feels she would like to incorporate that into her action plan.

Box 6.1: Brainstorming guidelines to use when following up with patients

1. The patient identifies a problem (write the problem down for the patient to see).

2. Ask the patient to list possible solutions.

3. Request that the patient not analyze the solutions during the brainstorming.

4. The patient should just throw out ideas that come to mind—no idea is stupid. Promote creativity when the patient is listing ideas.

5. Write the ideas down for the patient.

6. If you have additional ideas, ask the patient if you can add a couple of ideas to the list.

7. Ask the patient if he or she would like to try one of the ideas on the list.

Kate asks Jane to define her revised goal. Kate listens carefully, in case Jane needs some WHAT guidance. Once again, Kate asks Jane about her confidence level. Kate wants to make certain that Jane leaves with a well-defined goal she feels confident that she can accomplish.

Kate then arranges for a follow-up appointment with Jane. She also reaffirms the successes Jane had over the past 2 weeks and reinforces the reasons why Jane wants to make diet changes. This is a very important step. The reason to change needs to outweigh any of the barriers, and it will help keep the patient on the path to achieving a goal.

Review of the Goal-Setting Process

To review, here are the steps to use to help patients leave with an achievable and believable action plan:

1. Start your session with a patient with a question such as, "What is your biggest concern today?"

2. Guide your patient with open-ended questions, like "Tell me more...."

3. Use reflective listening—paraphrase and repeat back to the patient what he or she just told you.

4. Identify a change that is important to the patient, something he or she wants to do.

5. Next, make sure the patient leaves with an action plan based on the WHAT system.

6. Before the session ends, check the patient's confidence level on a scale of 0 to 10 (where 0 means there is no way that the patient feels he or she can accomplish the goal and 10 means the patient is absolutely certain that he or she will be successful).

You want your patient to have a confidence level of at least 7. If the confidence level is lower, guide the person toward revising the goal to make it more achievable.[6]

7. Arrange follow-up—it may be via e-mail, phone call, fax, or appointment—within the next 2 weeks.

Jane's Story (Part 3)

Let's work through another example with Jane. She wants to lose weight, and her RDN, Kate, aims to help her set a behavior goal that allows her to work toward her ultimate goal of weight loss. Remember, Jane needs to determine what she wants to work on. For weight loss, her goal will probably be linked to eating, drinking, or physical activity.

> **Kate:** Jane, you said you are concerned about your weight. You are upset with the 30 pounds you gained over the past 2 years, and you just mentioned that your doctor told you that the health problems you are having are linked to your weight gain. You told me your blood pressure is too high, and you now need two types of medications to control it. You also said that your blood sugar and cholesterol are going up. What is the one thing you want to do when you leave this office that will help you with your goal to lose weight and ultimately improve your health?

> **Jane:** I need to change my eating habits.

> **Kate:** What is one thing you want to do differently this week regarding your eating habits?

Jane: I eat too much after dinner.

Kate: It sounds like you want to eat less after dinner.

Jane: Yes—I want to stop eating snacks after dinner.

Kate: Okay, so your main focus will be not eating snacks after dinner. *(Note: Following the WHAT system, this first part of the discussion answers the questions of what Jane wants to do and when she wants to do it. Therefore, Kate moves on to how often Jane wants to skip evening snacks. Kate already set the time frame at 1 week.)* How many nights this week do you want to stop snacking?

Jane: Every night. I don't want to eat evening snacks at all. *(Note: When a patient reaches this point of defining a specific goal, you will want to check his or her confidence level.)*

Kate: Jane, on a scale of 0 to 10, zero being there is no way you can go without after-dinner snacks every day to 10 being absolutely certain you can skip after-dinner snacks every day, where are you? *(Note: It may be helpful to have a scale similar to Figure 6.1 for patients to use when setting their confidence level.)*

Jane: I think I'm at about 5. *(Note: Hearing this number, Kate sets out to do a little probing. She needs to help Jane increase her confidence level.)*

Kate: How many times a week do you have a snack after dinner?

Jane: Every night. *(Note: Going "cold turkey" seems like it is going to be too difficult for Jane. Often, setting a goal for 3 to 5 times a week is more realistic, but let your patient make that decision.)*

Kate: What changes could you make to your goal so your confidence level goes up to at least 7?

Jane: If I started with no snacks 2 times a week and had something healthy for a snack twice a week, then I would be at a 7.

Kate: Okay, for part of your goal, I hear that you want to go snack-free for 2 nights this week. Which evenings would you like to choose?

Jane: I take a pottery class on Monday night, so that would be a good night to skip a snack. My husband works late on Wednesday evening. That would be another good night to go snack-free.

Kate: You are choosing to skip your evening snack on Monday and Wednesday. Now, for the other part of your goal, which 2 evenings do you want to have healthier snacks, and what will those snacks be?

Jane: Friday night we go to the movies, so I will just have popcorn at the movie. Then I will have fresh veggies on Tuesday night. *(Note: Listening to Jane, Kate thinks about how many calories and how much fat are in movie popcorn.)*

Kate: May I offer you some suggestions on healthful snacks? *(Note: Kate is asking for permission before she offers her expert advice to Jane.)*

Jane: Sure, I need all the help I can get.

Kate: I have a handout here that lists some suggested choices for low-calorie, healthful snacks. You will notice that veggies are on here—great choice! Air-popped popcorn is also on the list. A 3-cup serving is only about 100 calories; you can also pop the corn in the microwave in a bag if you don't have an air popper. On this other handout, it lists some snack comparisons. You will notice that a small buttered popcorn at the movie theater is almost 600 calories. If you get it unbuttered, then it is about 350 calories. While popcorn can be a healthy low-calorie choice, you may want to consider how it is prepared, and how much you are going to have.

Jane: Wow. I didn't know movie theater popcorn has that many calories. I think I will skip the popcorn at the movie and make my own on Saturday night. Plus, this will save me some money!

Kate: To sum up, your plan is to be snack-free after dinner on Monday and Wednesday evenings. Then you plan to choose healthy, lower-calorie snacks after dinner twice a week—veggies on Tuesday and air-popped popcorn on Saturday night.

Jane: That is correct!

Kate: Let's check your confidence level again about your new snacking goal for this coming week. The scale starts at 0—as a reminder, that means you are 100% certain that you cannot achieve your goal. The other end of the scale is 10. At that end, you are absolutely certain that you can reach your goal of changing your snacking for four evenings this week. Where would you rate yourself, Jane?

Jane: I am ready to make some changes so that I can lose weight. This doesn't seem like a very hard first step, so I would rate myself at an 8.

Kate: Jane, that's great. You may want to write your goal for this week down and consider posting it somewhere at home, somewhere you would see it often. Also, logging your progress on evening snacking can be helpful.

Jane: That is a good idea. I will write it down right now and put it on my refrigerator when I get home. Then I will write down what I eat and drink every night after dinner.

Kate: The fridge door is where I post things that I want to remember too! And I also track goals I set for myself. I plan to meet with you a week from today at 2 pm.

Some of you may already be familiar with and use the SMART (specific, measurable, attainable, relevant, and time-based) system for goal setting. The concepts of SMART and WHAT goal setting are very similar. Use what works best for you or what you are most comfortable with.

Practice Exercises

Exercise 1

Practice helping your patients put the WHAT (or SMART) into their goal setting.

Exercise 2

Take the goal that you wrote down for yourself in Chapter 3, and put it into the WHAT (or SMART) format. Measure your confidence level and revise your goal if you are not at a 7 or higher. Consider setting your action plan for 1 week and track your progress. Write down your plan:

- *What* will you do? *When* will you do it? And *where*?
- *How much* or *how many*? And *how often*?
- Is your plan *achievable* and believable (use the confidence scale)?
- Your *time frame* is 1 week from today!

References

1. Norris SL, Lau J, Smith SJ, Schmid CH, Engelgau MM. Self-management education for adults with type 2 diabetes: a meta-analysis of the effect on glycemic control. *Diabetes Care.* 2002;25:1159-1171.

2. Renders CM, Valk GD, Griffin SJ, Wagner EH, Eijk VJ, Assendelft WJ. Intervention to improve the management of diabetes in primary care, outpatient and community settings: a systematic review. *Diabetes Care.* 2001;24:1821-1833.

3. Polonsky WH, Earles J, Smith S, et al. Integrating medical management with diabetes self-management training: a randomized control trial of the Diabetes Outpatient Intensive Treatment program. *Diabetes Care.* 2003;26:3048-3053.

4. Brown SA, Blozis SA, Kouzekanani K, Garcia AA, Winchell M, Hanis CL. Dosage effects of diabetes self-management education for Mexican Americans: the Starr County Border Health Initiative. *Diabetes Care.* 2005;28:527-532.

5. Bodenheimer T, Davis C, Holman H. Helping patients adopt healthier behaviors. *Clin Diabetes.* 2007;25:66-70.

6. Lorig K, Sobel D, Gonzalez V, Minor M. *Living a Healthy Life with Chronic Complications.* Boulder, CO: Bull Publishing; 2006.

Chapter 7:
When Patients Need More Than Nutrition Counseling

As an RDN, you will encounter patients who may or may not be ready to make lifestyle changes. Often, you may not fully understand the reasons why these patients are not open to change. In Chapter 1, we noted that all of us have worked with "noncompliant" patients (ie, patients who do not return for their follow-up appointments regardless of how hard we try to get them back). In Chapters 3 through 6, we explored several techniques to help us engage our patients. We discussed the importance of letting patients set the agenda and working with patients to ensure the goals they set are individualized and based on the lifestyle changes they want to make. Despite your best efforts, however, some patients still do not seem to be ready or able to make changes. What is going on with these patients?

Many health care professionals have experienced the frustration of working with patients who have chronic health care conditions but don't make positive behavior changes. What else do we need to explore to engage these patients? In 2001, the first Diabetes Attitudes, Wishes, and Needs (DAWN1) study looked at this question and reached some important conclusions.[1] This international cross-sectional study used questionnaires to explore how patients and health care professionals perceived diabetes and the stressors surrounding this disease. The study included 5,140 people who had either type 1 or type 2 diabetes, as well as 2,705 physicians and 112 nurses. Among the participants, only 19.4% of those with type 1 diabetes and 16.2% of those with type 2 diabetes indicated that they followed self-management recommendations set by their health care professionals.[1] These results support what we discussed in previous chapters: The choices people with chronic conditions make every day will have a much larger impact on their health and other medical outcomes than any decision the health care provider makes during a medical appointment.[2]

The DAWN1 study also explored the level of distress patients felt at the time of diagnosis, as well as several years after getting the diagnosis of diabetes. More than 85% of the participants reported high distress levels at the time of diagnosis. Even 15 years later, participants indicated that their treatment was too complicated, and one third stated they were tired of taking their medication. On the other hand, the study showed that many of the health care professionals were frustrated their patients did not follow their advice. They believed that many of their patients were not achieving desirable health outcomes and were experiencing devastating complications as a result of their noncompliance with recommended health care treatment.[1]

The results from the DAWN1 study have changed the way we work with individuals who have diabetes. Much more emphasis is being placed on the emotional distress experienced by our patients. A simple question—"What concerns you the most about your chronic disease?"—helps the health care professional explore that emotional distress.[3] Responses give us an insight into what is really bothering our patients and helps us determine whether they are ready to make lifestyle changes. When we ask this question, we might learn that a patient has difficulty adapting to or accepting the disease, family or work issues, or financial stressors. Many patients who are working on their lifestyle changes could increase their success level if they also receive appropriate emotional support from their family, friends, health care team, and others. Other patients may have mental health concerns, such as depression or anxiety, that make it difficult for them to focus on their health. In addition to affecting self-care, untreated mental health disorders can negatively affect relationships and job performance and elevate stress levels. Living with a mental health issue is also linked with increased alcohol and drug use and more difficulty following medical regimens.[4]

In 2013, the findings of the second DAWN study, named DAWN2 confirmed and deepened the understanding of how often people with diabetes are experiencing distress linked to having and managing their diabetes. It also surveyed and reported on how much diabetes affects family members. In addition, it showed how patient-centered care and support is not being adequately delivered in clinics and through health systems. The study was conducted in 17 countries and included 8,596 adults with diabetes. The results of DAWN2 showed that diabetes distress was still reported by 44.6% of the participants, but only 23.7% reported that their health care team asked them how diabetes affected their life.[5]

RDNs can play a very important role in helping patients with their health distress. When working with people who have chronic conditions, we need to be prepared to recognize potential mental health concerns and make the appropriate referrals. In this chapter, we discuss some of these conditions and explore assessment tools that will be helpful in your decision making. This chapter also provides ways to help patients whose self-management and health care are affected by financial constraints.

Mental and Emotional Health Issues

A report of the US surgeon general estimates that 1 in 5 Americans experience some type of mental health illness in any given year, and 2 out of 3 people with mental illness will not seek help.[4] According to Sederer and colleagues,[6] there is "overwhelming evidence that mental disorders and medical illnesses are strongly linked." They continue:

> Medical illnesses such as cardiovascular disease, diabetes, asthma, and cancer are associated with mental illnesses, and the more serious the medical condition, the more likely it is that the patient will experience a mental illness. Individuals with depressive disorders are about twice as likely to develop coronary artery disease, twice as likely to have a stroke, more than four times as likely to have a myocardial infarction (MI), and four times as likely to die within 6 months of an MI as people without depressive disorders. Depression is a common poststroke condition, and effective treatment of depression can improve cognitive functioning and survival. People with diabetes are two times as likely to have depression as the general population, and the presence of depression as a comorbidity to diabetes

is associated with poor adherence to medication regimens, greater complications of diabetes, increased numbers of emergency room visits, and poorer physical and mental functioning.

Clearly, the detection of possible mental health issues and appropriate referrals are very important. Have a plan in place to help patients who may have a mental illness. Set up lines of communication with the primary care providers so you can closely coordinate your efforts to identify patients' mental health concerns. For example, determine whether mental health screening will be a part of the primary care visit and/or explored by you.

Whether or not you screen patients, you should communicate any concerns about their mental health to the primary care practitioner. Addressing mental health concerns is a key step for your patients to achieve success when making lifestyle changes to maintain or improve their health outcomes.

One strategy to assist patients is to make available educational materials about stress, depression, and anxiety and where to get additional help. These materials increase awareness about the topics and enable your patients to know they can broach the topic with you.[7]

Depression

Since depression can be a common mental health problem, especially for people with chronic health conditions, it is particularly important that you have a plan in place for depression screening. Working with primary care providers is essential. Learn whether they regularly screen patients for depression. If they do, do you have access to the results of the assessment and the treatment plan?

If the primary care team does not routinely screen patients, determine how you can work together with the provider to develop a process for including depression screening as part of patient care. This process may include screening patients who concern you and referring them back to their primary care providers for a more detailed assessment and care. Another option may be to help the primary care offices develop and implement a plan to detect and treat depression in the clinics. This process may also require that this information be shared with you during the referral process.

Patient Health Questionnaires PHQ-2 and PHQ-9 are two tools used for depression screening.[8] The PHQ-2, shown in Figure 7.1, asks just two questions and is easy and quick to administer in any setting. It lets the RDN (or other health care provider) determine which patients would benefit from a more in-depth depression assessment and treatment, which is done or coordinated by the primary care provider. A "yes" answer to one or both of the questions on the PHQ-2 is considered a positive response and indicates that a person may have depression. However, it is not a perfect tool. Research indicates that this sort of quick screen may provide 5 false positives for every accurate positive response.[9] In addition, the PHQ-2 is best for identifying major depressive disorders and does not enable a practitioner to measure the impact of a person's depression on activities of daily living. A positive initial screen should be followed with more in-depth screening by a physician using a detailed tool like the

PHQ-9, shown in Figure 7.2 (pages 122–124).8 This helps the physician diagnose, treat, and monitor the severity of depression.

Figure 7.1: PHQ-2 Questionnaire

PHQ-2 Questionnaire for Major Depressive Disorders

During the past month:

Have you often been bothered by feeling down, depressed, or hopeless?

☐ Yes   ☐ No

Have you often been bothered by little interest or pleasure in doing things?

☐ Yes   ☐ No

NOTE: An affirmative answer to either question is a positive test result; a negative answer to both questions is a negative test result.

The PHQ-2 is adapted from the Primary Care Evaluation of Mental Disorders (PRIME-MD) developed by Spitzer, MD, Janet BW Williams, PhD, Kurt Kroenke, MD, MACP, and colleagues with an educational grant from Pfizer Inc. No permission is required to reproduce, translate, display, or distribute the patient health questionnaire (PHQ).

Figure 7.2: PHQ-9 checklist

Nine-Symptom Depression Checklist

Patient Health Questionnaire (PHQ-9)

Patient Name: _____

Date: _____

Over the <u>last 2 weeks</u>, how often have you been bothered by any of the following problems?

	Not at all	Several days	More than half the days	Nearly every day
1. Little interest or pleasure in doing things	☐	☐	☐	☐
2. Feeling down, depressed, or hopeless	☐	☐	☐	☐
3 Trouble falling/ staying asleep, sleeping too much	☐	☐	☐	☐
4. Feeling tired or having little energy	☐	☐	☐	☐
5. Poor appetite or overeating	☐	☐	☐	☐

	Not at all	Several days	More than half the days	Nearly every day
6. Feeling bad about yourself or that you are a failure or have let yourself or your family down	☐	☐	☐	☐
7. Trouble concentrating on things, such as reading the newspaper or watching television	☐	☐	☐	☐
8. Moving or speaking so slowly that other people could have noticed, or the opposite: being so fidgety or restless that you have been moving around a lot more than usual	☐	☐	☐	☐
9. Thoughts that you would be better off dead or of hurting yourself in some way	☐	☐	☐	☐

PHQ-9 Questionnaire for Depression
Scoring and Interpretation Guide
For physician use only

Scoring: Count the number (#) of boxes checked in a column. Multiply that number by the value indicated below, then add the subtotal to produce a total score. The possible range is 0–27. Use the table below to interpret the PHQ-9 score.

Not at all   (#) _____ × 0 = _____

Several days   (#) _____ × 1 = _____

More than half the days   (#) _____ × 2 = _____

Nearly every day   (#) _____ × 3 = _____

                              Total score: _____

Interpreting PHQ-9 Scores

Diagnosis	*Total Score*
Minimal depression	0–4
Mild depression	5–9
Moderate depression	10–14
Moderately severe depression	15–19
Severe depression	20–27

Action for Score

≤ 4	The score suggests the patient may not need depression treatment.
5–14	The physician uses clinical judgment about treatment, based on the patient's duration of symptoms and functional impairment.
> 14	The score warrants treatment for depression, using antidepressants, psychotherapy, and/or a combination of treatment.

The PHQ-9 is adapted from the Primary Care Evaluation of Mental Disorders (PRIME-MD) developed by Spitzer, MD, Janet BW Williams, PhD, Kurt Kroenke, MD, MACP, and colleagues with an educational grant from Pfizer Inc. No permission is required to reproduce, translate, display, or distribute the patient health questionnaire (PHQ).

Physicians and mental health professionals may also use other tools, such as the 21-question Beck Depression Inventory, to detect and measure the severity of depression. Additional depression screening tools currently in use include the Medical Outcomes Study Short Form (SF 20) and the Zung Self Rating Depression Scale, which is also available under different names.[10] These tools take more time to administer and may require more expertise in the field of depression than an RDN typically has.

A depression self-assessment method suggested by Lorig and colleagues in *Living a Healthy Life with Chronic Conditions* is for the patient to ask himself or herself what he or she does to have fun. If the person is unable to answer the question quickly, suspect that depression may be an issue for that person.[11]

If you are going to play a role in depression screening and you suspect a patient may have depression, you may broach the subject by mentioning to your patient, "Sometimes people have a lot of extra stress in their lives that may make it difficult to make healthful changes. This stress can be linked to having health problems, job or family issues, or financial concerns. When that is the case, extra help and sometimes medications can help people cope. I have a fast and simple screening tool [a self-assessment version of the PHQ-9] that can help identify whether a person would benefit from additional help or medication. I can help you go through it right now, if you are interested, or I can give you a copy to take home and look over. What would you like to do?" If the patient decides to take the tool home, recommend that he or she let you or the physician know what the assessment showed.

Ideally, the primary care practitioner takes the lead in the depression diagnosis and treatment. Current guidelines suggest the physician schedule a full diagnostic interview with a patient who has a positive depression screening.[12] In addition, the provider may also want to assess thyroid function, vitamin B-12 deficiency, sleep disorders, liver function, and other possible medical causes for signs of depression.

As we mentioned earlier in this chapter, if the primary care practitioner has not screened the patient for depression or if you suspect the patient may have a depression problem, it is appropriate for you to screen the patient. Referring the patient back to his or her practitioner and following up with the practitioner is crucial to make sure the patient is receiving a more detailed assessment and care, if indicated. When patients are screened for depression, it is critical to have support services in place.[7]

Patients with depressive disorders have successfully responded to short-term psychotherapy, with or without the addition of medication. Be prepared to reinforce medication regimens and discuss nutrition-related issues. For example, if medication is used, the patient will typically not see any effects on their mood for 2 to 6 weeks. However, patients often expect immediate results and may be disappointed if they do not know what will happen. If medications are prescribed, patients will also need to know that they should not stop their depression medication once they feel better. Stopping depression medication abruptly can worsen the symptoms. As an RDN, you can work with patients to remind them of this information and check to see whether they are using medications as prescribed. You may also be able to help patients with regular physical activity and stress-reduction techniques that are helpful in the management of depression.[9] In addition, some medications used to treat depression can affect appetite and weight status, and at least one drug should not be taken with certain foods. Your patients will benefit from knowledge of these drug-nutrient interactions.

Anxiety Disorders

Nearly one quarter of the population will be affected by an anxiety disorder at some time in their lives.[13] Anxiety disorders include panic disorder, agoraphobia, obsessive-compulsive disorder, and post-traumatic stress disorder. An overview of these and other types of panic disorders that tend to overwhelm patients and negatively affect their lives can be found on the Freedom from Fear website (www.freedomfromfear.org).

Many anxiety disorders are difficult to treat, as patients with anxiety disorders may also have alcoholism, depression, or suicidal thoughts. However, effectively dealing with anxiety disorders can also help with problems that patients have with substance abuse and depression.[13]

Anxiety is more common in people with eating disorders than in the general population. Individuals may experience anxiety before their eating disorder developed; anxiety may have even been present during childhood. (Eating disorders are discussed in greater detail later in this chapter.)

To identify anxiety in patients, you could ask as part of the assessment, "What concerns do you have about your condition?" If a patient has diabetes, you could suggest, "Tell me about the aspects of diabetes you worry about."[14] You could also use the GAD7 tool to screen for anxiety. A self-assessment version for patients is posted on the Patient website (www.patient.co.uk; from the Home page, search "GAD7"). Patients can click on "Generalized Anxiety Disorder Assessment Calculator" to perform a self-assessment.[15] Patients can also go to the Freedom from Fear website (www.freedomfromfear.org) and take an online screening test for anxiety or depression.

Health Distress

Another measure that may be useful, especially among your patients who have serious health conditions, is a measurement of health distress. Figure 7.3 shows a tool, called the Health Distress Scale, that Lorig and colleagues at Stanford University[16] adopted from the Medical Outcomes Study.[17] This tool can give you an idea of how much distress patients are feeling related to their illnesses or health conditions. Like depression or anxiety, patients may need additional treatment for health distress before they are able to effectively implement positive self-management strategies.

Eating Disorders

It is crucial to identify when a patient has a disordered eating condition and make referrals for additional assistance as indicated. The major classifications of eating disorders include the following:[18]

- Anorexia nervosa—The patient has an excessive self-push to become thin. Most will maintain a

Figure 7.3: Health distress scale used by Lorig and colleagues

These questions are about how you feel and how things have been with you during the past month. For each question in the chart below, please circle the number that comes closest to the way you have been feeling.

How much time during the past month...	None of the time	A little of the time	Some of the time	A good bit of the time	Most of the time	All of the time
1. Were you discouraged by your health problems?	0	1	2	3	4	5
2. Were you fearful about your future health?	0	1	2	3	4	5
3. Was your health a worry in your life?	0	1	2	3	4	5
4. Were you frustrated by your health problems?	0	1	2	3	4	5

Scoring: Score each item as the number circled. If two consecutive numbers are circled [for an item], score the higher (more distress) number. If the numbers [circled for an item] are not consecutive, do not score the item. The scale score is the mean of the 4 items. If more than one item is missing, set the value of the scale to missing. Scores range from 0 to 5; higher scores indicate more distress about health.

Adapted with permission from Stewart AL, Hays RD, Ware JE, Health perceptions, energy/fatigue, and health distress measures. In: Stewart AL, Ware JE. *Measuring Functioning and Well Being: The Medical Outcomes Study Approach*. Durham, NC: Duke University Press; 1992:143-172.

low body weight and show a deep level of concern with weight gain.

- Bulimia nervosa—The person does not seem to be able to control eating. Most overeat and then vomit, take laxatives, or exercise excessively. People with bulimia also show an exaggerated concern for being overweight.

- Other eating disorders—There are additional eating disorders that do not meet the criteria for anorexia or bulimia; they are referred to as eating disorders not otherwise specified (EDNOS).

The prevalence of eating disorders is unknown, as many people are secretive about their disordered eating. Young women between the ages of 18 and 30 years seem to be the group most affected by disordered eating. Men can also have eating disorders, with gay men having a potentially higher risk than heterosexual men. Athletes (both male and female) also seem to be affected by eating disorders; bulimia is the most common type of eating disorder among athletes. Individuals who want to lose weight and seek help toward this end are the most likely population to have disordered eating. As many as 50% of people interested in losing weight may have an eating disorder.[18]

Individuals with an excessive concern about weight and body shape, those with poor self-esteem, and those with a history of sexual abuse or other traumatic experiences are more likely to develop eating disorders.[17] In addition, other psychiatric disorders are often linked with eating disorders.

One screening tool that is available to help people identify their risk of having an eating disorder is the anonymous interactive tool provided by the National

Eating Disorders Association (www.mybodyscreening .org). It may be information that you can have available for patients you work with. In addition, it has been recommended that providers use the SCOFF questionnaire to help identify those who may have eating disorders. It includes these questions:

- Sick—Do you make yourself sick or vomit after a meal because you feel uncomfortably full?
- Control—Do you fear loss of control over how much you eat?
- One stone—Has the patient lost 14 lbs in a 3-month period?
- Fat—Do you believe you are fat even when others tell you that you are too thin?
- Food—Does food dominate your life?[19]

Patients who answer "yes" to two or more of the questions are at high risk for having an eating disorder (bulimia or anorexia nervosa). A more comprehensive evaluation and referral for care are recommended in these cases. Working with providers and the health care system to screen for eating disorders and making certain that care is in place to treat eating disorders are critical for addressing conditions that can potentially be deadly.

Patients with eating disorders can benefit greatly from the services of a treatment team that includes a mental health specialist as well as an RDN. Some patients may need medications to treat the eating disorder or other mental health disorders (such as post-traumatic stress disorder or obsessive-compulsive disorder). Depending on the severity of their eating disorder, some may also benefit from an inpatient program.

Medical nutrition therapy is also an essential component of treatment. In its position statement on nutrition intervention in the treatment of anorexia nervosa, bulimia nervosa, and other eating disorders, the Academy of Nutrition and Dietetics reinforces the role of the RDN in helping to develop a nutrition plan in coordination with the patient with an eating disorder as well as other team members. Ideally, the RDN then establishes an ongoing relationship with the patient to help with the achievement of treatment and nutrition-related goals. When working with patients with eating disorders, RDNs will benefit from having enhanced knowledge of behavioral health care.[18]

Financial Concerns

Some patients may not share their financial concerns with members of their health care team. For example, they may take less medication than prescribed or be unable to purchase healthful foods because of financial constraints. They may also live in areas with limited local resources, such as grocery stores or pharmacies, or lack means of transportation. Consider asking patients whether money concerns have ever caused them to delay or not follow medical care recommendations. A simple question to ask is, "Do you have trouble paying for…?" Or you could say, "Some of my patients have had trouble paying for some of their medications. Has that happened to you?" If you find that a patient has financial concerns, a referral to a medical social worker may help the person access programs that assist with medical and health care expenses.

You can also provide helpful information to patients on local free or low-cost services. Some of these services might include the following:

- clinics and hospitals with sliding scales,
- medication assistance programs,
- Medicaid programs,
- Veteran's Administration programs,
- senior services provided through your area agency on aging or local senior centers,
- organizations specific to certain conditions (eg, Arthritis Foundation, American Diabetes Association, National Kidney Foundation),
- religious institutions (such as the Catholic Diocese or Lutheran Social Services) and social service organizations,
- local federally qualified health centers,
- health department services, and
- food pantries.

Recognize your limitations as you seek to assist others—you will not be able to help every person who walks through your door. Sometimes, other health care professionals or different services are a priority for the patient. Do what you can to screen patients and make appropriate referrals to other sources of help. When patients address mental health, family issues, and financial concerns, they often move closer toward being able to work with you on health-behavior changes.

Practice Exercises

Exercise 1

Do you and other health care providers with whom you work have a process in place to assess patients for mental health concerns? If yes, what is the process? If not, how can you help put something into place?

Exercise 2

Are adequate resources in place to address mental health conditions in your community? If not, do you have ideas on how your community and health system(s) might enhance the services that are available?

References

1. Funnell M. The Diabetes Attitudes, Wishes, and Needs (DAWN) study. *Clin Diabetes*. 2006;24:154-155.

2. Rubin RR, Anderson RM, Funnell MM. Collaborative diabetes care. *Pract Diabetol*. 2002;21:29-32.

3. Anderson RM, Funnell MM. *Diabetes Concerns Assessment Form*. Ann Arbor, MI: Michigan Diabetes Research and Training Center, University of Michigan; 2005.

4. Office of the US Surgeon General. Mental health: a report of the surgeon general. http://www.surgeongeneral.gov /library/mentalhealth/home.html. Published 1999. Accessed June 7, 2015.

5. Nicolucci A, Kovacs B, Holt RIG, et al. Diabetes Attitudes, Wishes and Needs second study (DAWN2): Cross-national benchmarking of diabetes-related psychosocial outcomes for people with diabetes. *Diabet Med*. 2013:30:767-777.

6. Sederer LI, Silver L, McVeigh KH, Levy J. Integrating care for medical and mental illnesses. *Prev Chronic Dis*. 2006;3(2):A33. http://www.cdc.gov/PCD/issues/2006 /apr/05_0214.htm. Accessed June 7, 2015.

7. US Preventive Services Task Force. Screening for depression in adults. http://www.uspreventive servicestaskforce.org/uspstf09/adultdepression/addeprrs .htm. Released December 2009. Accessed June 7, 2015.

8. Ebell MH. Screening instruments for depression. *Am J Family Med*. 2008;78:244-246.

9. Arrol B, Khim N, Kerse N. Screening for depression in primary care with two verbally asked questions: cross sectional study. *BMJ*. 2003;327:1144-1146.

10. Halstenson C, Brunzell C. Depression, celiac disease, and cystic fibrosis. In: Ross T, Boucher J, O'Connell B. *Diabetes Medical Nutrition Therapy and Education*. Chicago, IL: American Dietetic Association; 2005:146-156.

11. Lorig K, Holman H, Sobel D, Laurent D, Gonzalez V, Minor M. *Living a Healthy Life with Chronic Conditions*. 3rd ed. Boulder, CO: Bull Publishing; 2006.

12. Putting prevention into practice: an evidence based approach. *Am Fam Physician.* 2003;67:1561-1562. http://www.aafp.org/afp/2003/0401/p1561.html. Accessed June 7, 2015.

13. Freedom from Fear website. http://www.freedomfromfear.org. Accessed June 7, 2015.

14. American Association of Diabetes Educators. *The Art and Science of Diabetes Self-Management Education: A Desk Reference for Health Care Professionals.* Chicago, IL: American Association of Diabetes Educators; 2006.

15. Generalised anxiety disorder assessment. http://patient.info/doctor/generalised-anxiety-disorder-assessment-gad-7. Accessed June 7, 2015.

16. Stanford Patient Education Research Center. Health distress. http://patienteducation.stanford.edu/research/healthdistress.html. Accessed June 7, 2015.

17. Stewart AL, Hays RD, Ware JE. Health perceptions, energy/fatigue, and health distress measures. In: Stewart AL, Ware JE. *Measuring Functioning and Well Being: The Medical Outcomes Study Approach.* Durham, NC: Duke University Press; 1992 :143-172.

18. Position of the American Dietetic Association: Nutrition intervention in the treatment of anorexia nervosa, bulimia nervosa, and other eating disorders. *J Am Diet Assoc.* 2006;106:2074-2082.

19. Luck AJ, Morgan JF, Reid F, et al. The SCOFF questionnaire and clinical interview for eating disorders in general practice: comparative study. *Br Med J.* 2002;325(7367):755-756.

Chapter 8:
Alternative Approaches That Assist with Behavior Change

In addition to what has been discussed in this book so far, there are other tools and techniques, such as meditation, prayer, expressive writing, and humor, that we can share with our patients as they work on changing their behavior. These tools may help to reduce stress, anxiety, and depression and enhance calmness and relaxation. When our patients can deal more effectively with emotional or health distress, they will often feel better, sleep more restfully, and be more able and willing to make behavior changes to improve their health. Reducing stress may also have other clinically meaningful outcomes through the lowering of the body's inflammatory response. While not a substitute for medical care, your patients may find one or more of these techniques useful in helping to address their health concerns.

Meditation

> *Breathing in, I calm my body. Breathing out, I smile. Dwelling in the present moment, I know this is a wonderful moment.*
>
> —*Thích Nâh´t Hạnh*

Meditation, as a practice, is thousands of years old and is frequently associated with Buddhism. In the past 40 years, the use of meditation has become more common as a way to assist with stress reduction and relaxation. A 2014 review of the research surrounding mindfulness meditation showed that it helped reduce anxiety, depression, and pain.[1] Studies conducted at the Cousins Center for Psychoneuroimmunology at UCLA have indicated that meditation can help reduce stress, depression, and anxiety and assist in the treatment of insomnia.[2] In addition, the Ornish program for reversing heart disease includes stress management techniques as one of the treatment modalities.[3] Meditation programs can be found in hundreds of hospital systems across the US, through community-based organizations, and at universities.

Some of the different meditation techniques include the following:[4]

- Visualization/guided imagery—This is a method where the person mentally takes himself or herself to a peaceful place such as a beach or a spot in the woods and concentrates on the sights, sounds, and smells. Some may use a teacher/guide or a taped program to help with the visualization.
- Mantra meditation—In this form of meditation, the person generally sits quietly and repeats a word or a phrase to help calm distracting thoughts.
- Transcendental meditation (TM)—In TM, each person is given an individualized mantra and silently repeats it in a given way.
- Mindfulness meditation—This type of meditation consists of becoming aware of one's present state. The person may focus on his or her breathing and

let thoughts pass through his or her mind without judging or contemplating them.

- Other practices that may include meditation are Qigong and tai chi. Some types of yoga also include a meditative portion.

These are some suggestions for getting started with meditation:

- Find a comfortable place, sit quietly for at least 5 to 10 minutes to start, breathe, and repeat a mantra or word. Some people find it helpful to also play some relaxing music.
- Try online meditation. Here are a few resources:
    ◦ UCLA Mindfulness Awareness Research Center (http://marc.ucla.edu/body.cfm?id =22)
    ◦ Ronald Siegel, PsyD, assistant professor at Harvard Medical School (www.mindfulness -solution.com)
    ◦ Anne and Dean Ornish, MD (https:// www.youtube.com/playlist?list=PL5CFE 57A8962E76B7)
- Join a meditation group. In addition to Buddhist temples, other organizations are embracing meditation for the health and wellness benefits. Check your local institutions including:
    ◦ hospitals,
    ◦ community centers, and
    ◦ universities.

- Get a phone app—for example, the Mayo Clinic Meditation app uses a clinically validated method of meditation.

Deep Breathing

The key to long life is to keep breathing.

—*George Burns*

Studies indicate that deep breathing exercises can benefit almost everyone by helping to reduce stress, lower blood pressure, and slow the heart rate.[5] For example, deep breathing was part of a stress-reduction pilot program offered to first-year University of Toledo medical students in 2010; a total of 272 out of the 496 students participated in the 3-year study. One of the primary outcomes was that students became more aware of their stress and reported that they felt better equipped to handle it. Over 80% of the students were satisfied with the program and described it as having beneficial outcomes.[6] Deep breathing is also one of the techniques taught to participants of the Stanford Chronic Disease Self-Management Program, an evidence-based program designed to help people with chronic health conditions develop the skills needed to manage them. In addition, it was a method used by Harvard Medical School cardiologist Herbert Benson, MD, to invoke the relaxation response.

Deep breathing is a technique that can be used any time. For example, a person can stop and take a couple of deep breaths if feeling stressed and anxious. A person may also have one or two specific times during the day to practice breathing. The method as taught in the Stanford program is to put one hand on the upper chest and the other on the belly. Breathing in deeply through the nose, the person should feel the hand on the diaphragm move outward as the lungs fill will air. The person is then instructed to purse his or her lips and breathe out, and the hand on the belly will then move inward with the exhale.[7]

Gratitude

> In life, one has a choice to take one of two paths: to wait for some special day—or to celebrate each special day.
>
> —Rasheed Ogunlaru

Many times it is easy to focus on what we don't have or can't do. Some people with chronic or serious health conditions may spend a long time grieving over the loss of their health and over the changes that they have to endure. Helping them make an effort to focus on what they can still do and on other things in their lives for which they are grateful may help them have a more positive outlook and feel happier; however, ruling out or treating depression or health distress may also be needed.

A study that involved 65 people with neuromuscular disease randomized participants to either gratitude or control groups. Each person completed a daily subjective life appraisal as part of the study; in addition, the gratitude group listed what they were grateful for each day. The participants in the gratitude group exhibited more positive feelings and fewer negative experiences throughout the study than the control group. In addition, the gratitude group reported an improvement in sleeping and a higher quality of sleep, as well as an enhancement in well-being. Spouses and significant others of the gratitude participants confirmed the improvement in well-being that the participants reported.[8]

Other benefits of focusing on what we are grateful for include the following:

- being more connected to others (Those who focus on their blessings seem to reach out and help others more often.);[8]
- strengthening the relationship a person has with his or her partner, especially when the focus of gratitude is on the positive things that the partner has done for the person;[9]
- improving heart health; and
- strengthening the immune system.

Here are some things your patients can try to expand their use of being grateful.[10]

- Keep a gratitude journal. It may be helpful for them to choose a time each day to write down what they are grateful for. They may decide to write down one or more things every day. Just like goal setting, your patients may want to be specific about what they appreciate. Instead of writing "I am grateful for my husband," for example, a patient could write, "Since getting sick, I appreciate the extra things my husband now does for me, like grocery shopping, cooking, and laundry." It may also be helpful to find the positive in what can be viewed as negative experiences. If someone has diabetes-related complications and needs additional medical treatment, a positive thing may be that the patient has the health care team, technology, and medications to treat this new health issue.

- Notice the good in life throughout the day.
- Give at least one compliment each day. It may be telling someone something you appreciate about him or her, or you may mention something you are grateful for, such as, "Thank you for helping me to be more active by getting up and walking with me 3 mornings this week."
- Commit to no complaining, gossiping, or criticizing for 10 days.
- Give time or money to a cause or organization that you believe in.

Positive Thinking

The last of human freedoms—the ability to chose one's attitude in a given set of circumstances.

—*Viktor E. Frankl*

Many people suffering from the loss of their health are unable to do some or many of the things they used to be able to do, and they may find it easy to view their lives in a negative way. Many healthy people also look at what is wrong in their lives and what they don't have. While feeling grateful is part of positive thinking, finding ways to reframe life experiences that are often viewed negatively may also help our health.

Positive self-talk/thinking has been linked to a variety of health benefits:[11]

- living longer,
- being able to cope with difficulties of life better,
- lowering risk of death from heart disease,
- experiencing less depression and distress, and
- having better mental and physical health.

While researchers don't know why people who use positive thinking/self-talk see the health benefits listed above, it is speculated that they may deal with stress more effectively. Being more relaxed may also help them maintain healthier lifestyles.

The Stanford Chronic Disease Self-Management Program also includes positive thinking as one of the techniques people can use to help them better manage their health conditions. Here are some things people can do to overcome negative thoughts:[7]

- Write down some negative thoughts you have had recently.
- Think about how to change them into positive thoughts.
- Write down your new, positive thoughts.
- For 1 day, try to identify when a negative thought comes into your mind. Immediately change it into a positive thought. Use your written positive thoughts to help you, if needed.
- Continue to practice changing negative into positive.

Following are a few examples of changing negative self-talk into positive self-talk:

> **Negative:** I will never be able to keep weight off; I am stuck in a cycle of losing and gaining.
>
> **Positive:** I have been successful at losing weight many times. I just need to learn some new strategies to keep the weight off.

> **Negative:** I don't have enough time to exercise.
>
> **Positive:** I can start to be more active by finding 10 to 15 minutes each day to go for a walk.

> **Negative:** It is too hard to change how I eat.
>
> **Positive:** I can find one way to eat better this week.

Expressive Writing

> *Writing about stressful situations is one of the easiest ways for people to release the negative effects of stress from their bodies and their lives.*
>
> —*James Pennebaker, PhD*

Did you know that the simple act of writing down your thoughts and feelings for a few days may have significant health benefits? Expressive writing has helped improve outcomes for older adults who have had surgery. It has also helped patients lower medication doses, improve blood pressure and cardiac symptoms in those who have a heart attack, and control symptoms of asthma or rheumatoid arthritis.

First studied by James Pennebaker, PhD, expressive writing can benefit one's health and help people stay healthy. In the short term, people using expressive writing techniques show an increase in distress, negative mood, and physical symptoms when compared to controls. However, at longer-term follow-up, many studies have reported health improvements:[12]

- reduced blood pressure,
- improved mood,
- enhanced feelings of well-being,
- fewer depressive symptoms,
- less frequent hospitalizations, and
- improved health function.

Other benefits include missing work less often, improved memory, better sports performance, and, for students, higher grade point averages. However, expressive writing hasn't been shown to improve diets or get people more physically active.[13]

All types of people have been shown to benefit from expressive writing. Men tend to experience more positive changes than women from using writing. In addition, people who tend to have more aggressive and hostile personalities are helped more by writing than those people who are naturally more easygoing and open.[13] Also, expressive writing may be especially helpful for those with asthma, rheumatoid arthritis, HIV, pain, or sleep difficulties.[12]

In using expressive writing, Pennebaker suggests that you write about the following:[14]

- what keeps you up at night—what is bothering you today—and

- traumas that are present in your mind—there is no need to dig up repressed memories.

Pennebaker also has guidance for how and when to write:[14]

- Write for about 20 minutes, 3 or 4 days in a row— that is the protocol that almost all studies on writing have used.

- Write more often, if that is what you feel you want to do.

- You may need to wait several weeks before you can write about a trauma in your life. Check in with yourself on how you feel about writing about a recent trauma.

- Make certain you have time to commit to writing.

- Try to write at about the same time each day and allow some time to reflect about what you have written.

- If writing about a particular trauma in your life seems to be too much for you to handle, don't write about it. Write about something else.

- Write nonstop during the 20 minutes and ignore grammar and spelling—it is meant only for you to look at.

- It is common to experience some sadness for a couple of days after writing.

- Write about an issue again in the future if you are feeling bothered by it. As a "booster shot," you may find that you don't need to write for 20 minutes over 4 days.

Box 8.1 outlines Pennebaker and Evans's guidance for those who want to try out expressive writing.

Expressive writing is not the same as journaling. For one thing, journaling may not yield the same health benefits as expressive writing. Those differences may be due to a variety of factors. While expressive writing has specific guidelines, journaling may not come with any detailed guidance. In addition, journaling may become rote and some may write about the same event numerous times. Also, depending on how journaling is used, it may not examine the feelings and emotions a person experiences in response to a stressor or traumatic event.

Talking about a trauma to another person may be better than writing about it if the person reacts favorably to what you are telling him or her. However, if the person has a negative reaction toward the disclosure, talking will actually be worse than writing. The same is true of reading what you have written to another person—if you don't get a positive reaction, you will end up feeling worse. Writing to and for yourself can have great benefits; there are even studies that suggest using the Internet to facilitate expressive writing is effective.[14]

These are some tips on how your patients can try out expressive writing:

1. Read the book by Pennebaker and Evans, *Expressive Writing: Words That Heal*. It has easy-to-read guidance for using expressive writing.

2. Identify counselors in your area who use writing as part of their treatment or see if they know of online expressive writing programs.

3. Become familiar with expressive writing and share details about it with your patients.

4. Use Box 8.1 as guidance for expressive writing.

Box 8.1: Instructions for expressive writing[14]

Day 1: Write about your deepest thoughts and feelings regarding a stressor or past trauma in your life. Explore how other people have been connected to the trauma and how it currently affects your life. How has this event or stressor impacted who you were in the past, who you are today, and what you would like to be like in the future?

Day 1 reflection: For each of the 4 questions, use a 0 though 10 scale where 0 means not at all, 5 means somewhat, and 10 means a great deal.

- How well did you express your deepest thoughts and feelings?

- How sad or upset are you?

- How happy do you feel?
- How valuable was your writing for you today?

- Describe how easy or difficult your writing was for you today.

Day 2: Look even more closely at your deepest thoughts and feelings. Write about the same trauma or choose another one. Use the same guidance provided for Day 1.

Day 2 reflection: Use the same questions from Day 1.

- How did writing go on Day 2 as compared to Day 1?

- Are you starting to see things differently?

Day 3: You can choose to write about the same issue(s) you wrote about on Day 1 or Day 2. In your writing today, focus on how your life is being impacted by the thoughts and emotions that are associated with the trauma or stressors you have experienced.

Day 3 reflection: Use the same questions that you used on Day 1.

Try to compare what you have written on the 3 days. What issues are coming to the surface most often? Has your writing brought out any new thoughts?

Day 4: Once again, explore your deepest thoughts and feelings about an experience you have had. Take a moment to think and then write about all that you have written. What have you lost, gained, or learned as a result of the trauma/stress you experienced? How will your past events help guide your actions and how you think in the future?

Day 4 reflection: Same as Day 1.

The last day of writing is often the most enjoyable for people. This practice can help them move past their trauma or stressors. Some may want to review all 4 days of writing, but it is advised that you wait for at least 2 or 3 days.

In their book *Expressive Writing: Words That Heal*, Pennebaker and Evans offer additional advice for ways to review your writing and determine if the writing has made a difference in your life.

Humor

> *The art of medicine consists of keeping the patient amused while nature heals the disease.*
>
> —*Voltaire*

Research has been done on whether laughter truly is the best medicine, but results have been mixed—and it is a tricky thing to study. Early laughter research used only male subjects and the sample sizes were small. Also, our knowledge of immunology was limited, using tests of immune function change in research was expensive, and few dollars were available to pay for laughter research.[15] More recently, there have been a few studies that looked at stress hormone release and laughter, but the results have also been mixed. Looking at a variety of other immune function markers has also yielded inconsistent results.[16]

There have been a few positive laughter studies published recently. One of them involved older adults. When compared with a control group, it showed that older adults who watched a short funny video had improvements in short-term memory and an increased capacity to learn. The study group also showed a drop in the cortisol level in their saliva from the beginning to the end of the humorous video; the control group had no change in the cortisol levels of their saliva.[17] Another study looked at pain tolerance and laughter. What the researchers found was that after their bout of laughter, the people in the laughter group showed a higher pain tolerance than the control group.[18]

Suggestions on ways for patients to put more humor into their lives include the following:[19]

- hanging funny cartoons or pictures in their homes or offices,
- keeping a stash of humorous movies or programs to watch when they need a laugh,
- finding humor in everyday life,
- spending time with people who make them laugh, and
- checking out joke books to find ones that tickle their funny bone.

Distraction

> *At painful times, when composition is impossible and reading is not enough, grammars and dictionaries are excellent for distraction.*
>
> *—Elizabeth Barrett Browning*

Some of the techniques outlined in this chapter may work because they serve as distractions. Getting the mind busy doing or thinking about other things can help with pain control, stress reduction, anxiety, and insomnia.[7] Other ways people may distract themselves include these:

- getting involved in a hobby, such as painting or woodworking,
- phoning or visiting a friend
- reading a book or watching a movie,
- getting some physical activity, or
- playing games in your mind, like naming a town for each letter of the alphabet.

Prayer

> *The function of prayer is not to influence God, but rather to change the nature of the one who prays.*
>
> —*Søren Kierkegaard*

If people you work with express a spiritual side, prayer may be used as a way to help support them making a behavior change. A Harvard Medical School study indicated that about 30% of adults used prayer in addition to conventional medical treatments for some of their health-related concerns, and 70% of those who used prayer reported that it was very helpful.[20]

Prayer may be like meditation for some and invoke a relaxation response. It may also help a person develop positive emotions; work by other researchers has indicated that positive emotions can cause physiological changes that lead to improved health.

Spirituality and religion are very personal and may be vastly different from person to person. As medical professionals, we don't want to push prayer or our religious beliefs onto patients. However, if prayer is part of their personal practices, we can support their use of prayer as an adjunct to conventional treatment.

Summary

We hope that this chapter has provided you with some additional tools and techniques that you can offer your patients who are having difficulty living with their chronic or lifelong health conditions. Of course, all should be assessed and treated for depression or health distress, if present. As mentioned previously, none of these are designed to be a replacement for other medical treatments. Rather, they are a supplement to the patients' current medical care.

Practice Exercises

Exercise 1

Choose at least one technique to try at home this week.

Reflect on how you felt as a result of using the technique.

Exercise 2

Share one or more techniques with a patient who is having difficult emotions linked to his or her health issues.

Follow up with the patient on the use of the technique and find out if it was helpful and in what way.

References

1. Goyal M, Singh S, Sibinga EMS, et al. Meditation programs for psychological stress and well-being. *JAMA Intern Med.* 2014;174(3):357-368. doi:10.1001 /jamainternmed.2013.13018.

2. Norman Cousins Center for Psychoneuroimmunology at UCLA website. http://www.semel.ucla.edu/cousins. Accessed on April 12, 2015.

3. Ornish Lifestyle Medicine. Stress management. http:// ornishspectrum.com/proven-program/stress -management/. Accessed on April 12, 2015.

4. Mayo Clinic. Meditation: a simple, fast way to reduce stress. http://www.mayoclinic.org/tests-procedures/meditation /in-depth/meditation/art-20045858. Published July 19, 2014. Accessed on April 12, 2015.

5. Harvard Health Publications, Harvard Medical School. Relaxation techniques: breath control helps quell errant stress response. http://www.health.harvard.edu/mind -and-mood/relaxation-techniques-breath-control-helps -quell-errant-stress-response. Published January 25, 2016. Accessed on April 15, 2015.

6. Brennan J, McGrady A, Lynch DJ, Wheartly K. Stress management interventions for first year medical students. *Annals of Beh Sc and Med Ed.* 2010;16(2);15-19. http:// absame.org/annals/ojs/index.php/annals/article /viewFile/23/23. Accessed on April 15, 2015.

7. Lorig K, Holman H, Sobel D. *Living a Healthy Life with Chronic Conditions.* Boulder, CO: Bull Publishing; 2014.

8. Emmons RA, McCullough ME. Counting blessings versus burdens: an experimental investigation of gratitude and subjective well-being in daily life. *Journal of Personality and Social Psychology.* 2003;84(2):377-389. http://greatergood. berkeley.edu/pdfs/GratitudePDFs/6Emmons -BlessingsBurdens.pdf. Accessed on April 22, 2015.

9. Mitchell RA. *Thankful Couples: Examining Gratitude and Marital Happiness at the Dyadic Level* [thesis]. Wilmington, NC: Department of Psychology, University of North Carolina Wilmington; 2010. http://dl.uncw.edu/etd/2010-1 /mitchellr/robynmitchell.pdf. Accessed on April 22, 2015.

10. Unstuck: a practical guide to gratitude. http://www .unstuck.com/gratitude.html. Accessed on April 22, 2015.

11. Mayo Clinic. Positive thinking: stop negative self-talk to reduce stress. http://www.mayoclinic.org/healthy-lifestyle /stress-management/in-depth/positive-thinking/art -20043950. Published March 4, 2014. Accessed on May 11, 2015.

12. Norelli LJ, Harju SK. Behavioral approaches to pain management in the elderly. *Clin Geriatr Med.* 2008;24:335-344.

13. Balkie K, Wilhelm K. Emotional and physical health benefits of expressive writing. *Adv Psychiatr Treat.* 2005;11(5):338-346. http://apt.rcpsych.org/content/11/5/338.full. Accessed on April 23, 2015.

14. Pennebaker JW, Kiecolt-Glaser JK, Glaser R. Disclosure of traumas and immune function: health implications for psychotherapy. *J Consult Clin Psychol.* 1988;56:239-245.

15. Pennebaker JW, Evans JF. *Expressive Writing: Words That Heal.* Eunumclaw, WA: Idyll Arbor; 2014.

16. Bennett MP, Lengacher C. Humor and laughter may influence health III: laughter and health outcomes 2008. *Evid Based Complement Alternat Med.* 2008;5(1):37-40. http:// www.ncbi.nlm.nih.gov/pmc/articles/PMC2249748/.

17. Bennett MP, Lengacher C. Humor and laughter may influence health IV: laughter and health outcomes 2009. *Evid Based Complement Alternat Med.* 2009;6(2):159-164. http:// www.ncbi.nlm.nih.gov/pmc/articles/PMC2686627/.

18. Bains G, Berk L, Daher N, et al. Effectiveness of humor on short-term memory function and cortisol levels in age matched elderly and diabetic subjects vs. control group–conference presentation. *FASEB J.* 2014;28(1).

19.   Dunbar RIM, Baron R, Frangou A, et al. Social laughter is correlated with an elevated pain threshold. *Proc Ro Soc London B Biol Sci.* http://rspb.royalsocietypublishing.org/content/early/2011/09/12/rspb.2011.1373.full. Published September 14, 2011. Accessed on May 11, 2015.

20.   Jantos M, Kiat H. Prayer as medicine: how much have we learned? MJA. 2007;186:S51-S53. http://faithhealth.wpengine.netdna-cdn.com/wp-content/uploads/2008/02/prayer-as-medicine-how-much-have-we-learned-mja-vol-186-num-10-may-21-2007.pdf. Accessed on April 15, 2015.

Chapter 9:
Building Long-Term Support
for Patients

In the previous chapters, you learned about evidence- and research-based patient counseling techniques, such as empowerment, motivational interviewing, and reflective listening, and explored ways to implement these techniques in your own practice. At this point, you are better prepared to work with those surly patients who come in with the attitude of a strong willed 2-year-old (or teenager or spouse) and are only interested in doing things their way. (You know the ones—they may sit with their arms crossed and make statements like, "I don't want to exercise, I don't want to start eating broccoli, and I am certainly not going to give up my beer and cigarettes!")

Maybe your patients are not yet doing everything that you and their other health care providers think they should do to manage their health conditions. Remember, making lifestyle changes and setting goals is not really about what we believe our patients should be doing but about what they are willing to change. As long as your patients are doing something positive, that is what counts. When you help them identify the lifestyle changes they want to make and then work with them to develop achievable goals, your patients build self-confidence. By assisting them with problem solving and developing relapse-prevention plans, you help them to manage their behavior change over time and in a variety of circumstances. As the old saying goes, success breeds success. How you work with patients on their first goal will set the stage for success or failure with future goals. And the approaches you use *are* helping your patients choose success!

As your patients make lifestyle changes that involve doing things differently, day after day, they will need long-term support. You are part of that support team, but even when you see patients once a week or twice a month, they are still on their own 99% of the time. You won't be with them at the grocery store or when they eat out. You aren't there at 6 AM to get them out of bed for a walk, and you can't police nighttime eating. What are some options for ongoing support?

Options for Ongoing Support

Continued Individual Sessions

You can continue to support patients over the long term through individual meetings, or you can link with them via technology, such as telephone, e-mail, videoconferencing, or web-based support. You already helped them get to this point. Therefore, you have shown that you have effective clinical and counseling skills. There is every reason to believe that ongoing contact with you will continue to work for your patients. In fact, the Academy of Nutrition and Dietetics Evidence Analysis Library documents the benefits of ongoing interaction with an registered dietitian nutritionist (RDN). Several studies have indicated that the more time people spent with RDNs, the more their low-density lipoprotein (LDL) and total cholesterol levels dropped.[1] However, questions about long-term support inevitably arise: What methods will you use to provide the support, and how will it be paid for? And will you have enough time to help all of the people who need long-term support?

Registered Dietitian Nutritionist–Led Group Sessions

Group sessions can be more time- and cost-effective than individual sessions, and they offer the benefit of people learning from and supporting each other. Group sessions are also part of the patient-centered medical home (PCMH) and are covered as part of the PCMH services provided by an RDN.

In three studies that looked at the effectiveness of group vs individual sessions to target weight loss or diabetes management in middle-aged subjects, the group sessions were *more* effective in the short term than the individual sessions.[2-4] More studies are needed, however.

One of the studies that looked at weight loss in overweight or obese premenopausal women also offered meal replacements in two of the arms of the study.[2] All participants attended 26 sessions over a 1-year period. The most successful group was led by an RDN and incorporated two meal replacements each day, and each participant lost an average of 9.1 pounds. The other arms included an RDN-led group with no meal replacement (4.1 pounds lost) and a physician office–based intervention, with meal replacements and individual visits with the doctor and nurse (4.3 pounds lost). Participants in the RDN-led group with meal replacement also had significantly more health improvements (lowering of blood pressure, cholesterol, triglycerides, and blood glucose levels) than the other two groups.

A 3-month study in Canada compared individual nutrition counseling with one-on-one sessions that were coupled with group education in adults with type 2 diabetes.[4] Participants in the group sessions had significantly greater adherence to nutrition recommendations, identified that they felt like they had more control over their eating, and exhibited a higher level of intention to make diet changes.

Another short-term (3-month) study also looked at weight loss.[3] Participants in the group therapy had significantly greater weight loss than those who participated in only the individual counseling.

While there isn't necessarily an optimal time identified for how many group sessions are needed to help make behavior change like weight loss, the Diabetes Prevention Program study, which has been a very successful study targeting weight loss to prevent type 2 diabetes, has been adapted to be offered as group sessions for people at risk to develop diabetes. It is a yearlong intervention, which begins with 16 weekly 1-hour sessions and then monthly meetings for the next 8 months.

People can and do ask for health care–related advice from peers, family members, and even total strangers. One of the authors recently chatted with an employee at a gas station convenience store, who mentioned that a customer with diabetes asked her for advice about which of the store's food items were diabetes-friendly. The employee was not sure what to tell him. After that encounter, she called one of the authors for advice, as she wanted to be able to help future shoppers and not give out any harmful or bad advice. It seems incredible that a person with diabetes would think that a convenience store employee would also be trained to provide expert nutrition advice, but it happens. And with the proliferation of information (or misinformation) on the Internet, even more advice from unlikely or untrained people is available.

Peer Support

That we humans can help each other is one of our unique human capacities.

—*Martin Luther King Jr*

Some forms of peer support may be largely unstructured, such as friend-to-friend help offered on an individual basis. Some support groups may also operate with very little structure. It is difficult to judge how helpful these various relationships and groups are, but it seems that some patients might benefit from such support. Some peer programs involve lay health education and support, whereas others do not.

Other peer-mentoring programs are more structured. One example is Alcoholics Anonymous. It involves a 12-step program in which alcoholics offer peer support to one another as they go through the steps. This model has been adapted for other health-related concerns, such as overeating. Some of the more structured peer-led support programs can be effective at helping those with health issues initiate positive behavior change.

The Robert Wood Johnson Foundation has financed a variety of programs to pilot ways to enhance community-based support for people with diabetes. For example, Move More, a free peer-to-peer program in Maine, trained lay volunteers to give support to people with type 2 diabetes who desired to get more physically active. Mentees also received pedometers, a nutrition and physical activity guide, and information about indoor and outdoor walking areas. Move More effectively built a network of 40 volunteers who supported people in getting more physically active using a variety of methods.[5]

Some diabetes self-management programs have been using *promotoras* (trained lay leaders) to teach diabetes education classes in some Spanish-speaking communities. Another of the Robert Wood Johnson diabetes initiatives in Texas evaluated the use of *promotoras* in teaching diabetes classes. They were trained to teach a 10-week series of classes, followed by 10 weekly support group meetings and weekly phone follow-up. Patients had improvements in metabolic control that were sustained over time.[6]

Another structured program that offers peer support is the Stanford Chronic Disease Self-Management Program. Designed to help people with chronic conditions, all potential leaders go through 4 days of training and practice teaching to become certified to lead the program. The program was designed to use lay leaders who also live with chronic health conditions. It is cofacilitated by two trained leaders, and a scripted manual helps guide the leaders through the six workshops that make up this program. One of the basic parts of the program is helping participants set and achieve goals each week. A study that followed 1,000 patients in the program for 3 years showed that participants were more active, reported less health distress, and saved health care dollars.[7]

Some weight-loss programs, such as Weight Watchers and TOPS (Take Off Pounds Sensibly), use peers to help and support each other. Tsai and Wadden systematically reviewed the effectiveness of these weight-loss programs and others.[8] Unfortunately, the authors were not able to identify many well-designed studies that examined different weight-loss programs. Weight Watchers had the best published data of any of the commercial or e-diet programs. In Weight Watchers, participants lost an estimated 10% of their body weight and were maintaining 3% of that weight loss after 2 years.

Technology Support

> Getting information off the Internet is like taking a drink from a fire hydrant.
>
> —Mitchell Kapor

This is the age of technology support, whether it is provided by you, other health care providers, family, friends, or online communities. Technology-based methods of communication, including phone, fax, videoconferencing, e-mail, and text messaging, are always evolving. More recent additions include instant messaging, blogs, Twitter, Facebook, or other social media to connect with our patients. Webinars and videoconferences are commonly used to help deliver our messages, and support is available through automated phone calls or smartphone applications. It is critical to stay up-to-date on emerging technological trends to help you connect more effectively with your patients.

Electronic Medical Records

Some of the patient support that technology can offer health care professionals starts with the electronic medical record (EMR). In 2005, a rapid adoption of health system EMRs was projected to save the US $81 million. Instead, we have seen our annual health care bill increase by $800 million. We have seen slow adoption of EMR systems, many are difficult to use, care and support processes are not always in place in the systems, and, in many instances, the patient does not have access to the data in his or her EMR.[9]

Although there have been some difficulties with EMRs, they will likely continue to be used and developed. Being part of a team that looks at EMR design, implementation, and improvement puts you in a position to help improve EMRs. It also allows you to voice your concerns and ideas about EMRs. HealthIT.gov offers guidance for implementing EMRs if you don't yet have a system in place or if you are upgrading what is currently in use.[10] In addition, CMS-funded Quality Improvement Organizations (QIOs) may be able to offer assistance in using an EMR more effectively. You can find your QIO on the American Health Quality Association website (www.ahqa.org/quality-improvement-organizations/whats-next-for-qios).

The use of EMRs, along with other health information technology, is an important part of the patient-centered medical home. It helps patients to be part of the team, better informed, and more engaged in their health. The EMR also assists with a better means of communication among all the team members and improves overall care to the patient.

Interactive Technology

Coupling health care with direct support to patients through technology has some distinctive advantages compared to using personal contact as the only means of support. It is possible for health care providers to program computers to make calls or send e-mails to follow up with patients who may have a chronic disease and/or depression. Using technology in this capacity eliminates the possibility of a person forgetting or getting too busy to make follow-up calls. In addition, it offers more privacy and anonymity, which can be especially important for those dealing with intensely private issues like substance or sexual abuse. Another important benefit of using technology to help support patients is that technology can be used to more easily expand outreach to a large numbers of people.[11]

While health care providers can use technology to deliver information quickly and easily, this might not be enough to inspire behavior change. The passive delivery may help to educate people, but it will not necessarily motivate people to make changes.[12] According to BJ Fogg, PhD, who directs the Persuasive Technology Lab at Stanford University, technology-based techniques that facilitate behavior change work best when they are interactive and are adjusted as the situation evolves. Interactive technology can be effective in these circumstances:

- The program leads the person through a series of steps to identify personal barriers to self-care such as taking medication regularly, being more active, or eating better. eDiets is an example of an online weight-loss program that poses questions to find out more about its customers. Based on the answers, eDiets offers audiotape programs to help people address diet concerns such as eating in response to stress.

- The technology involves simulations that allow people to practice new or different behaviors. One simulation program is the Nintendo game named *Bronkie the Brochiasaurus.* This interactive game has been shown to help kids with asthma better manage their condition.

- The technology takes on the role of a knowledgeable and supportive health counselor. MyDietitian is an example of using technology to link people with nutrition professionals for assistance with making eating changes.

- Certain online programs seem to benefit from being interactive. Internet-based weight-loss programs have proliferated; for example, Weight Watchers has an online version. (See Appendix for a list and description of additional online programs.) One study recently compared an online weight-control program to one that also included weekly behavior counseling e-mails and feedback from a counselor. Participants in both groups were at risk of developing type 2 diabetes and had started the program with a face-to-face meeting. All participated in the same Internet weight-loss program and all were instructed to submit their weights weekly. Adding the weekly e-mail and feedback to the Internet approach significantly improved weight loss over the yearlong program (4.4 kg vs 2.0 kg).[13]

Videoconferencing

Videoconferencing (interactive TV) has been tested as a means of delivering diabetes self-management education.

In one study, it was as effective as in-person classes. The videoconference participants rated the classes as helpful as the in-person class participants did, and both groups experienced similar reductions in stress.[14]

Texting health messages has also proliferated recently. When you consider that in 2013, 90% of US adults owned a mobile phone (56% owned a smartphone), 78% of teens owned a mobile phone (37% owned a smartphone), and texting was the most common use of cell phones (following phone calls), it is not a surprise that health issues are being influenced through text messaging. Looking at age differences, 97% those who are aged 18 to 29 use text messaging, while only 35% of those over the age of 65 use text messages. One study even indicated that those who are on Medicaid (79%) use text messaging more often than those who are uninsured (63%) or privately insured (65% to 68%).[15]

A variety of positive health changes have been identified in randomized controlled trials that use health texting. In an environmental scan conducted by the Department of Health and Human Services, eight out of nine studies that used text messaging found positive improvements in weight loss, smoking cessation, or diabetes management. One study found that blood glucose monitoring and control improved more through the use of text messages than through Internet monitoring. Two studies did not use tailored messages, and both showed a higher dropout rate than those with text messages that used tailored messages.[15]

Text messaging has also been used to increase the number of people who receive flu or pneumococcal vaccinations. In addition, those with depressive symptoms showed greater improvements in functional health and returned to employment or became employed at faster rates than participants who did not get text messages. Text messages to teens with severe asthma resulted in better adherence to medication protocols and a decrease in ER visits and missed school.[15]

As a means of behavior-change support, text messaging has been effective in interventions involving youth and adults. In addition, different ethnic groups and people from various income levels have been helped though the use of text messages. This may be a behavior-change support venue that is worthy of more research and expanded use of.[15]

Mobile Applications ("Apps")

Smartphones have become commonplace, and app use makes up 80% of consumer smartphone usage. Keeping up with this trend, it is estimated that there are several thousand health-related apps now available for download and use on smartphones, tablets, and computers. Dieting, weight loss, and fitness apps are found to be the most frequently downloaded of these health apps.[16] There are so many of these apps available that users can truly home in on monitoring what is important to them—whether it is calorie counting, nutrient adequacy, blood glucose monitoring, exercise, hydration, sleep patterns, or depression. It's important for RDNs to be aware of this trend and familiar with the most popular options to help clients integrate apps with their health care goals in a safe and effective way.

Users have cited many benefits to using health and fitness apps. They feel comfortable using their smartphones in public to input data, as it is fairly discreet. They also enjoy how fast and easy it is to input their data. According to one study, the average time a user took to check in was only 9.3 seconds.[16] Apps also often turn users' data into charts and graphs, providing visual feedback that makes it easy to see how close a user is to accomplishing his or her goal—or easy to see if he or she has fallen off track. Many apps feature games or competitions that help motivate users to continue with their progress, or they allow users to share their information with their friends or health care providers, including RDNs. Some apps also allow users to print or e-mail reports of their progress.

Some health apps have even been specifically created to help connect patients with RDNs. One example is MobileRD, which allows users to create a profile and submit concerns and daily data to RDNs for review and comment. To protect patient safety, they communicate via a secure e-mail system. By using this app, patients don't need to wait until their next appointment to receive feedback or support from their RDN. Another one of these apps is NuPlanit (www.nuplanit.com), which is being used in some hospitals, in academic settings, and by RDNs in private practice. Like MobileRD, the user can share info with the RDN. This app features interactive communication through video chatting and messaging.[17] However, it's important for users to realize—and as their RDN, you can remind them—that not all apps that claim to provide nutrition advice feature the support of actual RDNs. Users should review these kinds of apps carefully before beginning to use one.

With apps being fairly new to the table, a large amount of research has not been done on their effectiveness. But preliminary studies have shown that people who used health apps lost weight. However, it's important to note that in many of the studies, the smartphone apps were just one of the strategies used to address a particular issue. More rigorous randomized controlled studies are needed to truly evaluate the use of smartphones in assisting with health issues.[16]

Summary

Using Technology to Help Provide Behavior Change Support to Patients

You have many patients to serve, and helping them identify ways to get continued support with community resources or technology may enable them to sustain behavior changes over the long term.

There are several important factors to keep in mind regarding the use of technology. If your patients would like to use smartphone apps or websites to help them meet their goals, ideally the program should match the educational level, type and stage of disease or health condition, and attitude of each person.[11] By becoming familiar with different apps and programs that are available, you can suggest ones that you think would best benefit individual patients. This also helps eliminate the potential for unintended consequences to occur. For example, weight-loss diets aimed at the general public and readily available on the Internet may be harmful to some people who have other health concerns such as kidney disease. And, some apps or programs might include advice that may not be backed up by science. With so many patients using technology, and smartphones in particular, it's important to be able to guide them in the right direction.

With any technology-based support you plan to use, making sure that the privacy of the patient is protected is critical. Working with an IT person who has experience in Health Insurance Portability and Accountability Act (HIPAA) compliance can help ensure that your remote counseling sessions are kept private.

While some technology-based counseling— phone calls and videoconferencing—is covered by some insurance plans, most do not currently address mobile apps. Being aware of coverage by Medicare and the major health plans you work with will be important considerations when working with patients to choose ways to communicate.

See Box 9.1 (page 176) for tips on using technology in your practice. View the Appendix for a detailed list of different online programs and apps to help familiarize yourself with them.

Box 9.1: Tips for using technology in your practice

Read *Food & Nutrition Magazine* to stay updated on reviews of various health-and fitness-related apps.

Ask your patients how they prefer communicating in their personal lives. If they communicate primarily by text or e-mail, these might be good options for staying in contact with them between appointments.

Become familiar with popular apps. Your patients may be more apt to digitally track their habits using a mobile app if you have options to recommend.

Remember that if you use a specific app in your practice, it is the RDN's responsibility to ensure the app provider and its transmission programming are HIPAA compliant. Make sure to touch base with IT.

Encourage patients to share any knowledge or tips they've picked up from the health apps they use. You can confirm these tips, or help the patients customize them to best fit their specific needs and desires.

Charts and graphs in apps can show patterns in eating or exercise. Take a look at these to help your patients interpret *why* these patterns are occurring and how they can avoid any negative slumps.

Practice Exercises

Exercise 1

Identify the methods of long-term support you currently offer your patients, and find out about the community support programs that exist in your area. Are there any support groups that your patient population would benefit from?

Exercise 2

To assess what types of ongoing support your patients are receiving and what kinds of outcomes they are achieving, you may want to gather the following information:

- What percentage of your patients have access to ongoing support?
  - ° Do they use these services?
  - ° What types of outcomes do they have? How are you defining and measuring outcomes (eg, through the use of clinical data)?

- Do you have a data-tracking mechanism in place?

Exercise 3

Download a free food-tracking app of your choice, and use it as if you were a patient trying to achieve and maintain a certain amount of weight loss. Evaluate the benefits and challenges you experience while using the app. This exercise should help in interactions with patients who are also using apps.

References

1. Academy of Nutrition and Dietetics Evidence Analysis Library. The relationship between medical nutrition therapy (MNT) by a registered dietitian and patients' levels of dietary fat, saturated fat, serum cholesterol, and cardiac risk factors. http://www.adaevidencelibrary.com/evidence .cfm?evidence_summary_id=93. Accessed December 11, 2009.

2. Ashley JM, St. Jeor ST, Schrage JP, et al. Weight control in the physician's office. *Arch Internatl Med.* 2001;161:599-604.

3. Renjilian DA, Nezu A, Shermer RL, Perri MG, McKelvey WF, Anton SD. Individual versus group therapy for obesity: effects of matching participants to their treatment preferences. *J Consult Clin Psychol.* 2001;69:717-721.

4. Gucciardi E, DeMelo M, Lee R, Grace S. Assessment of two culturally competent diabetes education methods: individual vs. individual plus group education in Canadian Portuguese adults with type 2 diabetes. *Ethnic Health.* 2007;12:163-187.

5. Richert ML, Webb AJ, Morse NA, O'Toole ML, Brownson CA. Move More diabetes. *Diabetes Educ.* 2007;33(suppl 6):179S-184S.

6. Joshu CE, Rangel L, Garcia O, Brownson CA, O'Toole ML. Integration of a *promotora*-led self-management program into a system of care. *Diabetes Educ.* 2007;33(suppl 6):151S-158S.

7. Lorig KR, Ritter P, Stewart AL, et al. Chronic disease self-management program: 2-year health status and health care utilization outcomes. *Med Care.* 2001;39:1217-1223.

8. Tsai AG, Wadden TA. Systematic review: an evaluation of major commercial weight loss programs in the United States. *Ann Intern Med.* 2005;142:56-66.

9. Kellerman AL, Jones SS. Analysis & commentary: what it will take to achieve the as-yet-unfulfilled promises of health information technology. *Health Aff.* 2013;32:163-168.

10. HealthIT.gov. Providers and professionals. http://www
.healthit.gov/providers-professionals. Accessed June 10,
2015.

11. Fogg BF. *Persuasive Technology: Using Computers to
Change What We Think and Do.* San Francisco, CA: Morgan
Kaufmann Publishers; 2003.

12. Kennedy CM, Powell J, Payne TH, Ainsworth J, Boyd A,
Buchan I. Active assistance technology for health-related
behavior change: an interdisciplinary review. *J Med Internet
Res.* 2012;14(3):e80. http://www.ncbi.nlm.nih.gov/pmc
/articles/PMC3415065/. Accessed June 10, 2015.

13. Tate DF, Jackvony EH, Wing RR. Effects of Internet
behavioral counseling on weight loss in adults at risk for type
2 diabetes. *JAMA.* 2003;289:1833-1836.

14. Izquierdo RE, Knudson PE, Meyer S, Kearns J, Ploutz-
Snyder R, Weinstock RS. A comparison of diabetes education
administered through telemedicine versus in person diabetes
care. *Diabetes Educ.* 2003;26:1002-1007.

15. US Department of Health and Human Services. *Using
health text messages to improve consumer health knowledge,
behaviors, and outcomes: an environmental scan.* Rockville,
MD: US Department of Health and Human Services; 2014.
http://www.hrsa.gov/healthit/txt4tots/environmentalscan
.pdf. Accessed May 25, 2015.

16. Ventola CL. Mobile devices and apps for health care
professionals: uses and benefits. *PT.* 2014;39(5):356-364.
http://www.ncbi.nlm.nih.gov/pmc/articles/PMC4029126/.
Accessed May 25, 2015.

17. Stein K. Remote nutrition counseling: considerations in a
new channel for client communication. *J Acad Nutr Diet.*
2015;115(10):1561-1576.

Chapter 10:
Other Issues to Consider: Health Literacy, Cultural Diversity, and Biases in Health Care

In this book, we have discussed how to help patients make lifestyle changes and how various approaches will work in different scenarios. We also discussed certain barriers that you may encounter when working with patients, such as depression and other mental health issues and financial barriers to self-care (see Chapter 7). This chapter addresses selected other issues that you will want to consider when working with patients: health literacy, cultural diversity, and various biases, such as age or gender.

Health Literacy

Many of your patients may have low health literacy, and you might not even be aware of it! Health literacy is defined in *Health People 2010* as "the degree to which individuals have the capacity to obtain, process, and understand basic health information and services needed to make appropriate health decisions." Health literacy is more than a person's reading level. It also involves the ability to make what can be complex decisions based on what is read.[1] In fact, having low health literacy has been described as a silent epidemic—you can't always discover it just by looking at or talking with a person. Low health literacy can be found in patients of all income levels and across all races, ages, and backgrounds. According to the Institute of Medicine's report *Health Literacy: A Prescription to End Confusion,* nearly 50% of the US population has problems with health literacy, which lead to missed medical appointments, not taking prescriptions as directed, and misunderstanding other medical treatment.[2] According to the American Medical Association, low health literacy is "a stronger predictor of a person's health than age, income, employment status, education level, and race."[3]

Health literacy challenges may explain why some patients do not "comply" with certain requirements like reading food labels, following meal plans, taking medications, and filling out insurance forms. As you work to empower your patients, keep in mind that low health literacy may hinder their abilities to take charge of their health care.[2]

People with low health literacy are more likely to have chronic health conditions like diabetes, high blood pressure, or HIV/AIDS, and they manage these conditions less effectively than people with higher health literacy levels. In addition, they use more high-cost services to treat health conditions, like emergency room visits and hospitalizations, and they use fewer preventive health services such as flu shots and mammograms.[3]

Some US health care professionals mistakenly think health literacy mainly affects people who do not speak English or for whom English is a second language. In reality, only 15% of those who have limited health literacy were born outside the US.[2] While nonnative English speakers are at high risk for having low health literacy, so are older adults, people with low incomes, those who did not graduate high school, and racial and ethnic minorities.[4]

You may not immediately recognize that someone has limited health literacy, as people can develop ways to hide that they do not understand spoken directions or written materials, particularly if they feel ashamed or embarrassed about their literacy skills.[2] Fortunately, you can adopt a variety of techniques that will enhance your ability to communicate with patients who have health literacy concerns—remember, low health literacy is common! Keep in mind the following when working with a patient who has low health literacy:

- Speak slowly.
- Dump the medical terms. Keep your message simple. (For more help in using plain language, check out the Center for Plain Language website: www.centerforplainlanguage.org.)
- Watch for overload. Remember, the patient is in charge. If you want to give advice, ask for permission and offer just a couple of suggestions.
- Check back, or "close the loop." Did your patient understand the conversation exchange? Ask the person to explain to you what steps he or she is going to take. Make sure that you do not turn this into a test. Some experts in health literacy suggest that you start with something like, "I want to make certain that I am explaining things well. Taking medications in the right way can be very hard and confusing. Can you please tell me what changes we

made in your medications and how you are going to take them?"[5]

- Demonstrate whenever possible and allow patients the opportunity to practice. For example, label reading is a great opportunity to demonstrate and practice with a patient.

- Use handouts that also include pictures. Many studies have indicated that educational handouts and patient consent forms are difficult for many patients to read and comprehend. Recent research has indicated that Internet-based educational materials are also too difficult for many patients. Box 10.1 gives an overview of how to identify or develop patient forms and educational tools that more fully address health literacy concerns.[6]

Screening for Health Literacy

Some health care professionals believe that testing for health literacy may be demeaning to patients and prefer to use simple tools and words when working with *all* patients. However, others think that it may be helpful for one of the health care team members to assess each patient's health literacy.[2] Work with your health care partners to put in place a plan of action for your team. Will someone screen for health literacy? Will you play a role in screening?

Two reliable and easy-to-use tools that are used to evaluate health literacy are the Rapid Estimate of Adult Literacy in Medicine (REALM) and the Test of Functional Health Literacy in Adults (TOFHLA). With REALM, you provide a patient with a list of medical terms that are single syllable (eg, pill, stress) and multiple syllables (eg, inflammatory, potassium), and ask him or her to read the list. The test takes less than 5 minutes to administer and

Box 10.1: Developing patient-friendly handouts

- Limit information to one or two educational messages.

- Cover only items patients really need to know.

- Keep content at or below a sixth-grade reading level (SMOG and FRY are examples of two readability tests you can use to check the level).

- Use one- or two-syllable words.

- Avoid medical jargon.

- Use large font (at least 12 point) with upper- and lowercase letters.

- Make certain handouts have a lot of white space.

- Use bulleted items, as these are better than paragraphs.

- Use simple pictures.

score. The number of words that a person pronounces correctly helps identify his or her reading level. In addition, the test helps highlight some of the things the person may need help with, such as reading and following the directions on a prescription label.[2]

The Test of Functional Health Literacy in Adults (TOFHLA) is a two-part test that is available in English or Spanish. It poses a scenario for participants and then asks them to answer questions about the scenario. They are asked to fill in blank spaces from a multiple-choice list of answers. In addition to being a reading test, TOFHLA also poses numeracy questions, like figuring out how much medication to take and when to take it, based on looking at a drug label.

The Newest Vital Sign (NVS) is a quick and easy health literacy tool available in Spanish and English, which was designed for primary care.[7] Patients are given a health scenario and are then verbally asked a series of six questions. The entire screening can take less than 3 minutes. If a person answers four or more of the questions correctly, he or she probably does not have low health literacy. If the person answers fewer than four questions correctly, literacy issues are probably a concern. One NVS scenario of interest to RDNs is a nutrition-label scenario that requires people to do mathematical calculations (see Figures 10.1 and 10.2).

Additional Health Literacy Resources

In addition to the Center for Plain Language website (www.centerforplainlanguage.org), which we mentioned earlier in this chapter, there are many other excellent free or low-cost opportunities to improve your health literacy skills. For example, the Agency for Healthcare Research and Quality offers a Health Literacy Precautions Toolkit (http://www.ahrq.gov/professionals/quality -patient-safety/quality-resources/tools/literacy-toolkit /index.html).

To find more information on developing low-literacy print materials, check out this resource from the Centers for Disease Control and Prevention, called Simply Put (www.cdc.gov/healthliteracy/pdf/Simply_Put.pdf).

Figure 10.1: Newest Vital Sign nutrition label

Nutrition Facts		
Serving Size		½ cup
Servings per container		4
Amount per serving		
Calories 250	Fat Cal	120
		%DV
Total Fat 13g		20%
Sat Fat 9g		40%
Cholesterol 28mg		12%
Sodium 55mg		2%
Total Carbohydrate 30g		12%
Dietary Fiber 2g		
Sugars 23g		
Protein 4g		8%

*Percentage Daily Values (DV) are based on a 2,000 calorie diet. Your daily values may be higher or lower depending on your calorie needs.
Ingredients: Cream, Skim Milk, Liquid Sugar, Water, Egg Yolks, Brown Sugar, Milkfat, Peanut Oil, Sugar, Butter, Salt, Carrageenan, Vanilla Extract.

Figure 10.2: Score Sheet for Newest Vital Sign

Score Sheet for the Newest Vital Sign Questions and Answers

	ANSWER CORRECT?	
READ TO SUBJECT: This information is on the back of a container of a pint of ice cream.	**yes**	**no**

1. If you eat the entire container, how many calories will you eat?

   Answer: 1,000 is the only correct answer

2. If you are allowed to eat 60 grams of carbohydrates as a snack, how much ice cream could you have?

   Answer: Any of the following is correct: 1 cup (or any amount up to 1 cup), Half the container Note: If patient answers "two servings," ask "How much ice cream would that be if you were to measure it into a bowl."

3. Your doctor advises you to reduce the amount of saturated fat in your diet. You usually have 42 g of saturated fat each day, which includes one serving of ice cream. If you stop eating ice cream, how many grams of saturated fat would you be consuming each day?

   Answer: 33 is the only correct answer

4. If you usually eat 2500 calories in a day, what percentage of your daily value of calories will you be eating if you eat one serving?

   Answer: 10% is the only correct answer

READ TO SUBJECT: Pretend that you are allergic to the following substances: Penicillin, peanuts, latex gloves, and bee stings.

5. Is it safe for you to eat this ice cream?

   Answer: No

6. (Ask only if the patient responds "no" to question 5): Why not?

   Answer: Because it has peanut oil.

Interpretation   Number of correct answers:

Score of 0-1 suggests high likelihood (50% or more) of limited literacy
Score of 2-3 indicates the possibility of limited literacy.
Score of 4-6 almost always indicates adequate literacy.

Also, visit the website for the Pharmacy Health Literacy Center (http://pharmacyhealthliteracy.ahrq.gov/sites /PharmHealthLiteracy/default.aspx), developed by the Agency for Healthcare Research and Quality. You may get some useful tips in helping patients understand how and why to take medications. Resources you may want to check out regarding health literacy include the Institute of Medicine book *Health Literacy: A Prescription to End Confusion*[2] and the Pfizer Clear Health Communication Initiative (www.pfizerhealthliteracy.com).

Cultural and Ethnic Diversity

In earlier chapters, we discussed ways to identify patient priorities and use approaches like empowerment and motivational interviewing to help them refine goals. Having knowledge about and acceptance of food habits and the cultural beliefs of your clients can also be very important in building rapport and helping your patients set and make behavior changes.

When working with patients, learn about their cultural and ethnic backgrounds. Strive to understand and embrace cultural diversity. The following are some questions to consider as you work with patients from cultures different from yours:[2]

- Are there accepted gender norms, such as distinctive roles for men and women?
- Do extended family members play important roles in the patient's life or care?
- What traditional medicine beliefs or practices does the person embrace?

- What foods are accepted, celebrated, or forbidden?
- Do you need to consider culturally specific factors in counseling situations, like the appropriateness of eye contact or touching or the significance of body language?
- What are acceptable styles of dress?

As you consider these issues, remember to assess your patients as individuals—don't jump to conclusions about a specific patient's cultural practices based on general knowledge of that culture. Instead, ask culturally sensitive questions and observe personal behavior.

Use of Translators and Lay Health Workers

Depending on language skills, you may need to have a trained interpreter present to assist with medical terminology and concepts during discussions with your patients. In fact, the use of qualified interpreters is supported by the Americans with Disabilities Act. This includes making accommodations for those who are hearing impaired (ie, providing a sign language interpreter) or for those who speak a foreign language. For some patients, having lay health workers involved in care will also be valuable.

Additional Resources on Cultural Diversity

The Academy of Nutrition and Dietetics has a variety of resources that can help you work with clients who may come from different cultural backgrounds. For example, the book *Culturally Competent Dietetics: Increasing Awareness, Improving Care* is a collection of articles that were previously published in the *Journal of the Acad-*

emy of Nutrition and Dietetics. It offers practical advice from experts on ways to interact with people from other cultures. *The second edition of Spanish for the Nutrition Professional* explores cross-cultural communication techniques, teaches basic counseling phrases and vocabulary, and includes food pictures with their English and Spanish names. Another publication that is available is *Cultural Food Practices*, which includes guidance for working with 15 different cultures. You can purchase these books and review other resources on the Academy of Nutrition and Dietetics website (www.eatright.org).

Identifying and Addressing Biases

One of the authors has a 72-year-old friend, Mary. Recently, Mary went to a sporting goods store to purchase a new pair of racing cross-country skis. Despite her spry physical condition and ability to tell the shop salesperson what she wanted, the clerk, according to Mary, tried to steer her away from the racing skis. Mary felt this was a prime case of age discrimination. If the store clerk had gone out on the trails with Mary, he would have seen that her stamina and skill level were perfectly suited for racing skis. In the end, he did not deter Mary from buying the racing skis, either!

Mary persevered in her goals despite the clerk's apparent bias. However, in health care, practitioner biases can have notable consequences for the quality of care that patients receive. Although we all wish to consider ourselves personally free of bias, it is advisable to periodically reflect on these issues and how your perceptions of patients may be shaped by your assumptions about factors such as age, gender, weight, race, or ethnicity.

Age and Gender Bias

Age and gender discrimination have been documented in health care. A UK study involving more than 15,500 people who had been diagnosed with ischemic heart disease found that women, especially women older than age 65 years, were not prescribed the recommended treatment at the same level received by men.[8] Another study used a series of videotaped vignettes to "test" how 256 primary care doctors (men and women) would care for different patients. The study participants were similar in age, class, and race. Some of the cases were presented as women and some as men. The biggest difference in treatment was linked to gender. Women across all scenarios were asked fewer questions, received fewer tests, and had fewer medications prescribed.[9]

Weight Bias

People with overweight or obesity may be subjected to bias or discriminatory health care practices. One study[10] examined potential weight bias in health care professionals who specialized in the management of obesity and concluded that these health care professionals exhibited a significant "anti-fat" bias. In addition, the health care professionals endorsed the stereotypes of overweight and obese patients being "lazy, stupid, and worthless." Finding bias in this group of health care professionals was particularly surprising, as they understand the complexities of being obese and realize it cannot be simply attributed to personal choices. Similar weight bias against overweight and obese patients has been identified in other health care professionals, too. Some have said they spend less time with obese patients and tend to order more tests. Others have stated they are repulsed by obese people and would prefer not to treat them.[10]

Obese women are less likely to obtain preventive services such as breast and pelvic exams, even though they see their physicians more often. In part, this is linked to the negative body image of many obese women and their reluctance to have their bodies examined. However, some health care providers do not encourage obese women to receive care, and some do not want to examine them.[10]

Racial and Ethnic Disparities and Biases

Racial and ethnic differences in health care have been reported. Several studies have indicated that much of the difference in care for racial and ethnic minorities is due to socioeconomic factors and insurance status. Those without insurance, who also tend to have a lower income, receive fewer medical services. When there are language barriers, care received is even more suboptimal.[11]

Cognitive and Physical Disability Biases and Disparities

Currently, 1 in 5 Americans have some type of disability related to mobility, cognition, and/or self- or independent care. While anyone may have a disability, they occur more commonly in women, older Americans, and racial and ethnic minorities. People with disabilities are also more likely to be obese, have cardiovascular disease, be smokers, and engage in little leisure-time activity. In addition, some disabilities will be very visual, while others may be less obvious.[12] Another disturbing fact is that people with disabilities, especially those with developmental disabilities, are subject to more acts of violence than those who do not have disabilities.[13]

One thing we can do right away is to start using appropriate terminology when talking with or about people who have disabilities. Box 10.2 shows some examples of terminology to use and language to avoid. An easy thing to keep in mind is that we are talking about people who have some type of condition, so always use *people* or *person* with a descriptor, and be certain the descriptor is not offensive. Instead of saying, "He is slow," you could say, "He has a developmental disability."

Box 10.2: Language to use when referring to people with disabilities[14]

Language to use	Language to avoid
Person with a disability	The disabled, handicapped
Person with a developmental, cognitive, or intellectual disability	Slow, simple, retarded, moronic, or special person
Person who uses a wheelchair	Wheelchair bound, confined to a wheelchair
Person with a physical disability	Deformed, lame, spastic, crippled
Person who has a communication disorder	Mute, dumb
Person with a seizure disorder	Epileptic

Another thing that needs to be addressed on a global level is access. Currently, one of the greatest barriers to care for people with disabilities is access. Here we have a population that has more problems with obesity and lower amounts of leisure activity, and they may have limited opportunities to be active. Observe when people have difficulty navigating their environment and also ask them what needs to happen to make the clinic, hospital, or community organizations and spaces more accessible. There are also resources and architects that can assist with universal design; they can provide an assessment and help to make changes to better serve those who have disabilities.

While the 1990 Americans with Disabilities Act helps to protect people with disabilities from discrimination, there continue to be inequities in health care for those with disabilities, including the following:[12]

- Risky behaviors like smoking are less likely to be addressed in the clinic setting.
- Patients with breast cancer often recieve suboptimal treatment.
- There is an increase likelihood of death if diagnosed with lung cancer.
- Clinics and other centers for care are often inaccessible.

As with other groups, unconscious or conscious biases may be at play. Being aware of and addressing issues that affect people with disabilities is a first step. In addition, including people with disabilities, their families, and organizations that serve them would be beneficial in making changes to more effectively and humanely treat people who live with disabilities.

Additional Resources to Assess Potential Biases

Project Implicit has online mini assessments (Implicit Association Tests) on a variety of topics to help individuals and researchers look at conscious and unconscious preferences or biases for more than 90 different issues. Originally launched by Yale University as a demonstration website in 1998, Project Implicit has since grown into a research project overseen by four universities. It has been funded by the National Institute of Mental Health since 2003. A variety of information is provided on multiple websites.

- Project Implicit (www.projectimplicit.net) offers a general overview, news, and links to the other sites.
- Several assessments are available for people to complete (https://implicit.harvard.edu/implicit). Each assessment takes about 10 to 15 minutes. At the end of each assessment, participants are given feedback on preferences and potential biases.

Practice Exercises

Exercise 1

How does your practice address health literacy? What about the health care providers and systems you work with? Consider the following questions:

- Are your forms and educational tools patient friendly?
- Do you use teach-back skills and plain language and avoid patient overload?

If you answered "no" to these questions, what is one thing that you can begin implementing?

Exercise 2

What type of cultures or ethnic groups do you work with? If you have not already done so, consider taking time to learn more about their beliefs and practices, especially as linked to health and food.

References

1.   Glassman P. Health literacy. National Network of Libraries of Medicine. http://nnlm.gov/outreach/consumer/hlthlit .html. Accessed February 6, 2011.

2.   Institute of Medicine; Nielsen-Bohlman L, Panzer AM, Kindig DA, eds. *Health Literacy: A Prescription to End Confusion.* Washington, DC: National Academies Press; 2004. http://books.nap.edu/openbook.php?record _id=10883. Accessed June 27, 2010.

3.   Ad Hoc Committee on Health Literacy for the Council on Scientific Affairs, American Medical Association. Health literacy: report of the Council of Scientific Affairs. *JAMA.* 1999;281:552-557.

4.   US Department of Health and Human Services. Quick guide to health literacy. http://www.health.gov/communication /literacy/quickguide/factsliteracy.htm. Accessed November 20, 2009.

5.   Schillinger D, Piette J, Grumbach K, et al. Closing the loop: physician communication with diabetic patients who have low health literacy. *Arch Intern Med.* 2003;163:83-90.

6.   Weiss BD. Health literacy and patient safety: help patients understand. American Medical Association Foundation and American Medical Association; 2007. http://med.fsu.edu /userFiles/file/ahec_health_clinicians_manual.pdf. Accessed March 16, 2016.

7.   Weiss BD, May MZ, Martz W, et al. Quick assessment of literacy in primary care: the newest vital sign. *Ann Family Med.* 2005;3:514-522. http://www.annfammed.org/cgi /reprint/3/6/514. Accessed November 20, 2009.

8.   Williams D, Bennett K, Feely J. Evidence for an age and gender bias in the secondary prevention of ischaemic heart disease in primary care. *Br J Clin Pharmacol.* 2003;55:604-608.

9.   Arber S, McKinlay J, Adams A, Marceau L, O'Donnell A. Patient characteristics and inequalities in doctors' diagnostic and management strategies relating to CHD: a video-simulation experiment. *Soc Sci Med.* 2006;62:103-115.

10.   Schwartz B, Chambliss HO, Brownell KD, Blair SN, Billington C. Weight bias among health professionals specializing in obesity. *Obes Res.* 2003;11:1033-1039.

11.   Kirby JB, Taliaferro G, Zuvekas SH. Explaining racial and ethnic disparities in health care. *Med Care.* 2006;44:5. I64-I72.

12.   Iezzoni, LI. Eliminating health and health care disparities among the growing population of people with disabilities. *Health Affairs.* 2015;34(10):1947-1954. http://content.healthaffairs.org/content/30/10/1947.full. Accessed on October 29, 2015.

13.   Hughes K, Bellis MA, Wood, S, et al. Prevalence and risk of violence against adults with disabilities: a systematic review and meta-analysis of observational studies. *Lancet. 2012;*379:1621-1629.

14.   Centers for Disease Control and Prevention. Communicating with and about people with disabilities. http://www.cdc.gov/ncbddd/disabilityandhealth/pdf/disabilityposter_photos.pdf. Accessed on October 29, 2015.

Appendix:
Additional Resources

Chapter 2

Jortberg BT, Fleming MO. Registered dietitian nutritionists bring value to emerging health care delivery models. *J Acad Nutr Diet*. 2014;114:2017-2022.

Brown-Riggs C. The patient-centered medical home—the dietitian's role in this healthcare model that improves diabetes outcomes. *Today's Dietetian*. August 2012;14:26.

Committee on Quality of Health Care in America, Institute of Medicine. *Crossing the Quality Chasm: A New Health System for the 21st Century*. Washington, DC: National Academies Press; 2001. https://www.iom.edu/Reports/2001/Crossing-the-Quality-Chasm-A-New-Health-System-for-the-21st-Century.aspx.

Improving Chronic Illness Care. www.improvingchroniccare.org.

- Includes access to the Chronic Care Model

National Diabetes Education Program. Practice transformations for physicians and health care teams. http://betterdiabetescare.nih.gov.

Chapter 3

Anderson B, Funnel M. *The Art of Empowerment: Stories and Strategies for Diabetes Educators.* 2nd ed. Arlington, VA: Skelly Publishing; 2005.

- Order from the publisher (www.skellypublishing. com) or Amazon.com
- Available for 30 CPEs

Michigan Diabetes Research and Training Center. http:// diabetesresearch.med.umich.edu.

- Offers many books and tools on empowerment

Chapter 4

Prochaska JO, Norcross J, DiClemente C. *Changing for Good: A Revolutionary Six-Stage Program for Overcoming Bad Habits and Moving Your Life Positively Forward.* New York, NY: William Morrow and Company; 1994.

Chapter 5

Motivational interviewing . http://www.motivational interviewing.org/motivational-interviewing-resources.

- Includes motivational training, videos, and resources

Chapter 6

American Association of Diabetes Educators. AADE®7 System. www.diabeteseducator.org/Professional Resources/AADE7/A7S.html.

- Tool to help with patient goal setting and tracking

Lorig K, Holman H, Sobel D, Laurent D, Minor M. *Living a Healthy Life with Chronic Conditions*. Boulder, CO: Bull Publishing; 2012.

Chapter 7

Mental Health Concerns

American Dietetic Association. Position of the American Dietetic Association: nutrition intervention in the treatment of anorexia nervosa, bulimia nervosa, and other eating disorders. *J Am Diet Assoc*. 2006;106:2074-2082.

Freedom from Fear. www.freedomfromfear.org.

- Offers depression and anxiety self-assessment tools
- Made available by the National Nonprofit Mental Illness Advocacy Organization

Michigan Diabetes Research and Training Center. Diabetes concerns assessment forms. http://diabetesresearch.med.umich.edu/peripherals/profs/documents/emh/ConcernsAssessment.pdf.

- Other resources also offered

Patient Health Questionnaires (PHQ) Screeners. www
.phqscreeners.com.

- Free mental health disorder screening tools available for use by health care professionals
- Made available by Pfizer

Stanford Patient Education Research Center. Health
distress screening tool. http://patienteducation
.stanford.edu/research/healthdistress.html.

US Preventive Services Task Force. Recommendation
statement on screening for depression in adults.
http://www.uspreventiveservicestaskforce.org
/Page/Document/UpdateSummaryFinal/depression
-in-adults-screening1?ds=1&s=depression%20
screening.

Financial Concerns

Local service clubs and churches may be able to provide
short-term assistance, and many health systems also have
special programs for patients with financial concerns.

Centers for Medicare & Medicaid Services. Federally
Qualified Health Centers (FQHC). https://www.cms
.gov/center/fqhc.asp.

- FQHC provide sliding scale fees for many medical
services and medication

Disability.gov. https://www.disability.gov.

Indian Health Service. www.ihs.gov.

- Help for American Indians and Alaska Natives

National Council on Aging. https://www.ncoa.org
/audience/older-adults-caregivers-resources/.

- Resources for older Americans and their caregivers

Needy Meds. www.needymeds.org.

- Offers help with cost of medication

Salvation Army. www.salvationarmyusa.org.

- Offers temporary home, food, and medication assistance

Society of Saint Vincent de Paul: http://www.svdpusa.org.

- Offers temporary home, food, and medication assistance

US Department of Health and Human Services. www.hhs.gov.

- Links to health care questions and resources and special insurance for children

US Department of Veterans Affairs. www.va.gov.

- Additional help for veterans and widows of veterans.
- To check eligibility, go to www.va.gov/healthelig ibility/Library/tools/Quick_Eligibility_Check.

Chapter 8

Meditation

UCLA Mindfulness Awareness Research Center . http://marc.ucla.edu/body.cfm?id=22.

- Site has free audio-guided meditations available.

Siegel, R. www.mindfulness-solution.com.

- Audio meditation available

Preventative Medicine Research Institute. http://www.pmri.org/guided-meditations.html.

- Free audio meditations available

Expressive Writing

Pennebaker J, Evans J. *Expressive Writing: Words that Heal.* Enumclaw, WA: Idyll Arbor, Inc; 2014.

Distraction

Lorig K, Holman H, Sobel D. *Living a Healthy Life with Chronic Conditions.* Boulder, CO: Bull Publishing; 2012.

Humor

Mayo Clinic. Stress management. http://www.mayoclinic.org/healthy-lifestyle/stress-management/in-depth/stress-relief/art-20044456.

- Information about using laughter for stress management

Positive Thinking

Mayo Clinic. Positive thinking: stop negative self-talk to reduce stress. http://www.mayoclinic.org/healthy-lifestyle/stress-management/in-depth/positive-thinking/art-20043950.

Chapter 9

Diabetes Support

Better Choices Better Health for Diabetes. https://www
.ncoa.org/healthy-aging/chronic-disease/chronic
-disease-self-management-program/better-choices
-better-health/.

- Evidence-based program designed to help people with diabetes strengthen self-management skills

Children with Diabetes. www.childrenwithdiabetes.com.

- Online community for kids, families, and adults with diabetes

dLife Diabetes Support Forum. www.dlife.com/diabetes
-forum.

Diabetes Sisters. https://diabetessisters.org.

- Includes forum for women living with diabetes

National Diabetes Education Program. Diabetes health
sense. http://ndep.nih.gov/resources/diabetes
-healthsense/index.aspx.

- Offers resources devoted to supporting patient change, including searchable database of research, tools, and programs supporting patient behavior and lifestyle changes

Kidney Disease Support

DaVita. www.davita.com.

- Resources and support for those with kidney disease or those on dialysis

National Kidney Foundation. https://www.kidney.org
/patients

Weight-Loss Support

List below is only a partial list; many other plans are available.

Calorie King. www.calorieking.com.

- Food and exercise tracking, online support, and resources
- Fee charged

Diet.com. www.diet.com.

- Provides individualized menus for a variety of meal plans, fitness plans, live phone support, and online communities
- Fees charged for diet plan, support, and food

eDiets. www.ediets.com.

- Provides individualized menus for a variety of meal plans, fitness plans, live phone support, and online communities
- Prepackaged food available
- Fees charged for diet plan, support, and food

Jenny Craig. www.jennycraig.com.

- Program includes prepackaged foods
- Meeting or phone support available
- Fees charged for services

MyPlate. www.choosemyplate.gov.

- Resources and interactive tools, including personalized food plans and food tracker
- Free

Nutrisystem. www.nutrisystem.com.

- For-purchase meal replacement plan with online support

Overeaters Anonymous. www.oa.org.

- Support group based on the 12-step program
- Free

SparkPeople. www.sparkpeople.com.

- Free weight-loss and fitness website
- Includes food and exercise tracker, questions answered by registered dietitians and fitness experts, links with other people who are interested in weight loss, and a variety of resources

Take Off Pounds Sensibly (TOPS). www.tops.org/.

- Low-cost program that mainly provides support for weight-loss efforts of participants

Weight Watchers. www.weightwatchers.com.

- Online or phone and community meetings available
- Fees charged for services

Smartphone Applications for Weight-Loss Support

Below we have listed just a small sample of the many apps available; some apps charge fees.

Concrete Software. Fast Food Calorie Counter

Fresh Apps. Lose It! www.freshapps.com/lose-it.

My Fitness Pal. https://www.myfitnesspal.com.

- A fitness and calorie tracker

My Net Diary. www.mynetdiary.com.

- Includes a calorie counter that allows you to scan food bar codes for nutritional value

SparkPeople. www.sparkpeople.com/mobile-apps.asp.

- Free apps available for many smartphones

Weight Watchers Mobile.

- Participants can track their points

Chapter 10

Health Literacy Resources for Professionals

Agency for Healthcare Research and Quality. Pharmacy health literacy center. http://www.ahrq.gov /professionals/quality-patient-safety/pharmhealthlit.

- Resources and information related to health literacy and use of medications

Centers for Disease Control and Prevention. Simply put: a guide to creating easy-to- understand materials. http://www.cdc.gov/healthliteracy/pdf/Simply_Put .pdf

Health Resources and Services Administration. Health literacy. www.hrsa.gov/healthliteracy/default.htm.

- Variety of health literacy resources

National Patient Safety Foundation. Ask me 3. www.npsf. org/askme3.

- Resources to improve communication with patients who have low health literacy

The Pfizer Clear Health Communication Initiative. www
.pfizerhealthliteracy.com.

Assessment of Bias

Project Implicit. Implicit Association Tests. https://
implicit.harvard.edu/implicit.

- Online mini assessments on a variety of topics to
  help individuals and researchers look at conscious
  and unconscious preferences or biases for more
  than 90 different issues

Index

Page number followed by *b* indicates box; *f*, figure; *t*, table.